The
Irritable Bowel Syndrome
Sourcebook

The Irritable Bowel Syndrome Sourcebook

LAURA O'HARE

Contemporary Books

Chicago   New York   San Francisco   Lisbon   London   Madrid   Mexico City
Milan   New Delhi   San Juan   Seoul   Singapore   Sydney   Toronto

Library of Congress Cataloging-in-Publication Data

O'Hare, Laura.
    The irritable bowel syndrome sourcebook / by Laura O'Hare.
      p.   cm.
    Includes bibliographical references and index.
    ISBN 0-7373-0553-3
    1. Irritable colon—Popular works.   I. Title.

   RC862.I77 .O34   2001
   616.3'42—dc21   2001028568

Contemporary Books

A Division of The McGraw·Hill Companies

2 3 4 5 6 7 8 9 0 DOC/DOC 0 9 8 7 6 5 4 3 2

ISBN 0-7373-0553-3

This book was set in Sabon
Printed and bound by R. R. Donnelley—Crawfordsville

Cover design by Laurie Young
Interior design by Mary Ballachino/Merrimac Design

McGraw-Hill books are available at special quantity discounts to use as premiums and sales promotions, or for use in corporate training programs. For more information, please write to the Director of Special Sales, Professional Publishing, McGraw-Hill, Two Penn Plaza, New York, NY 10121-2298. Or contact your local bookstore.

This book is printed on acid-free paper.

CONTENTS

Part One: How IBS Occurs: Triggers and Effects / 1

Chapter One: The Digestive System and the Diagnosis / 3

Defining IBS / 4
How the Digestive System Works / 4
    The Stomach / 5
    The Small Intestine / 5
    The Large Intestine / 6
How Problems Arise / 7
    Gas / 7
    Cramping and Spasms / 8
    Diarrhea / 8
    Constipation / 9
IBS Distress and the Mind/Body Connection / 10
Differentiating Other Stomach Disorders / 11
Diagnostic Criteria for IBS / 14

**Chapter Two: The Connection Between
               Body and Mind / 17**

Stress / 17
    Hans Selye's Concept of Stress / 18
    Types of Stress / 19
    Stress Symptoms / 21
    IBS and Sensitivity to Stress / 22
    Stress Symptoms as a Cause of Stress / 23
Depression / 24
    Cause or Effect of IBS? / 24

Distinguishing Depression from Other
Feelings / 25
Types of Depression / 26
Therapy for Depression / 27

Chapter Three: The Female Factor / 31
Doctors' Attitudes / 32
IBS and Childhood Sexual Abuse / 34
Effects of the Menstrual Cycle / 37
The Disease to Please / 39

**Chapter Four: Disorders Commonly Linked
with IBS / 43**
Functional Disorders and IBS / 43
Fibromyalgia / 43
Nonulcer Dyspepsia / 46
Globus Hystericus / 47
Physical Disorders That May Trigger IBS / 48
Acute and Bacterial Gastroenteritis / 48
Alcohol Abuse or Dependence / 49
Food Allergies / 51
Food Intolerance / 53

**Part Two: How to Manage IBS:
Treatments and Strategies / 55**

Chapter Five: Diet Strategies / 57
Keeping a Food Diary / 57
Analyzing Your Diet Diary / 60
Common Trigger Foods / 60
Fats / 60
Dairy Products / 61

High-Fiber Foods / 61

Spices / 62

Caffeine / 62

Pinpointing Your Troublesome Foods / 63

What to Eat Instead / 65

Fast-Food Substitutions / 65

Breakfast / 65

Lunch and Dinner / 66

Delicatessen Substitutions / 67

Breakfast / 67

Lunch / 68

Pizza Parlor Substitutions / 68

Chicken and Other Entrée
  Takeout Substitutions / 69

Chinese Food Substitutions / 69

Mexican Food Substitutions / 70

Home-Cooked Meal Substitutions / 70

Breakfast / 70

Lunch / 71

Dinner / 71

The Right Environment for Eating / 72

Diet for Children with IBS / 73

Food Allergies / 74

Combating Fear of Food / 75

Reintroducing Foods in Your Diet / 76

Chapter Six: Stress Strategies / 79

Keeping a Stress Diary / 80

Ranking and Dealing with Stressors / 82

Easily Reduced Stressors / 82

Life's Little Irritants / 82

Household Chores and the
  Disease to Please / 85

Delegating / 86
Stress and Exercise / 88
    Yoga / 89
    Tai Chi Chuan / 90
    Exercise Classes and Workouts / 91
    Gardening / 91
    Playing with Children / 92
    Walking / 92
Stress and Psychotherapy / 95
Spirituality and Stress Management / 99
    Finding Help in Faith / 100
    Finding the Spiritual in Nature / 101
    Finding Help Through Prayer
        and Meditation / 102
Keeping Stress-Relievers Close at Hand / 105
    Humor / 106
    A Return to Childhood / 107
    Spiritual Reminders / 108

Chapter Seven: Alternative Therapies / 111
    Chinese Herbal Medicine / 111
    Acupuncture / 115
    Biofeedback / 115
    Hypnosis / 118
    Creative Visualization / 123

Chapter Eight: Medication Strategies / 125
    The Lotronex Fiasco / 125
    Croton lechleri: A Supplemental Option / 127
    Zelmac and Women with IBS / 129
    Antidepressants / 130
    Antibiotics / 131

Antispasmodics / 132
Antidiarrheals / 133
Over-the-Counter Medications / 133

Epilogue / 135

Further Resources / 139

Glossary / 143

Bibliography / 149

Index / 155

PART ONE

How IBS Occurs: Triggers and Effects

IF YOU ARE ONE OF THE MILLIONS around the world who have been diagnosed with irritable bowel syndrome (IBS), you are well aware that the diagnosis gives a name to your problem but no clear-cut solution. The search for a solution can be frustrating and disheartening. While quite a bit of information on IBS is available, much of it is not conclusive and may even appear contradictory at first glance. As I researched this subject—reading journal articles and books and reviewing relevant Web sites—I could imagine that many IBS sufferers, overwhelmed by the sheer glut of information, might throw up their hands, give up on a solution, and give in to IBS. If you are one, this book is for you.

The first part of the book, "How IBS Occurs: Triggers and Effects," describes how the digestive system functions, examines in detail the symptoms and triggers of IBS, and offers an overview of conditions that may be related to, or in some cases lead to, IBS.

The second part, "How to Manage IBS: Treatments and Strategies," addresses how you may develop individual ways to cope and live with IBS better—by making physical and mental adjustments in your daily life, from diet and exercise to psychotherapy and meditation.

I recommend that you first read the book with the goal of gathering general information, not answers. Aim to discover which elements of the IBS diagnosis—symptoms, triggers, and treatments—apply to you. Then consider which approaches might work best with your lifestyle and belief systems and what changes you'd be willing to make to feel better.

If I had to choose the most important idea you could take away from this book, it would be: *Handling IBS is a process that requires time and patience.* You didn't go to bed one night feeling terrific only to wake up the next day and discover that IBS had taken over your life. It will take time to get your life back. Before you decide that time is the one thing you don't have—and many of us feel that way these days—ask yourself these questions:

- How many hours do you spend worrying about, and recovering from, your bouts of IBS?
- How much of your productivity is diminished by IBS?
- How many days of work do you miss because of IBS?
- How is your quality of life affected by IBS?
- How much time with family and friends is lost to, or negatively affected by, IBS?

When you really think about it, you'll see how a small investment of time now can, and will, reap untold hours free of pain and discomfort. So take a deep breath, find a quiet place, and start down the road to taking care of yourself. Now is the time for you to begin living a life ruled by your heart and head, not your digestive tract.

To begin, learn what IBS is and is not.

CHAPTER ONE

The Digestive System and the Diagnosis

Irritable bowel syndrome (IBS) is a condition whose symptoms, triggers, and impact vary from patient to patient. Although the specific cause of IBS is still unknown, the impact of IBS is well documented. IBS affects up to 20 percent of the population, and the median age of sufferers is thirty-five. Although two-thirds of IBS patients are women, anyone can have the syndrome—including children.

A 1995 study, "Medical Costs in Community Subjects with Irritable Bowel Syndrome," targeted to white adults, estimated that this group of patients alone accounted for $8 billion per year in IBS-related medical costs. For some, IBS causes only discomfort; for others it is truly debilitating. Universally, the symptoms of IBS are matters that no one wants to discuss, let alone experience—pain, cramps, gas, bloating, diarrhea, constipation.

Just as the symptoms vary from sufferer to sufferer, so do the factors that trigger them. For one person it's fatty foods, for another raw vegetables. Some find themselves reacting to specific stressors; others feel that their symptoms come literally out of nowhere. The one common experience of IBS sufferers is frustration, for it is a condition with no clear-cut cause or cure.

Defining IBS

IBS is a *functional disorder,* a disorder diagnosed by its symptoms rather than by its specific physical cause. With IBS, the digestive system definitely reacts with a number of specific, and unpleasant, symptoms, but exactly what causes those reactions is unknown. To picture how your digestive system functions (or dysfunctions) in this way, imagine a similar disorder in your leg. The leg constantly aches and sometimes flares into pain. The doctor can find no pull, tear, bruise, or break; yet there is no question that something is wrong with the leg. Staying off the leg as much as possible, applying ice packs, exercising, and stretching eventually end, or at least greatly diminish, your symptoms. You are cured, or at least improved, without ever knowing what caused the problem. This is the journey you have to take to live better with IBS. Lacking a physical cause to address, you treat IBS by patiently and carefully identifying and treating its triggers and symptoms.

How the Digestive System Works

To understand some common causes of symptoms associated with IBS, it's important to know how your digestive (gastrointestinal) system functions. The gastrointestinal tract runs from the mouth to the anus. It is like a long tube whose cavity, or *lumen,* is surrounded by a wall that absorbs nutrients. The ability to absorb is heightened by the wall's surface of ridges and valleys, which expand the area that comes in contact with nutrients.

The gastrointestinal tract is sometimes separated, for discussion, into two parts—the upper GI tract and the lower GI tract. The upper tract includes everything above the large intestine; the lower tract includes the large intestine and everything below it.

The Stomach

The stomach is essentially a sack that sits beneath the diaphragm and under the rib cage. Its function is to hold food immediately after ingestion and to prepare it for digestion and absorption by the rest of the GI tract. The moment you see, smell, or eat food, your stomach relaxes and expands to be ready to take it in. When food arrives in the stomach, the stomach walls secrete acid, mucus, and pepsin, which mix with the food to ready it for the small intestine. Hydrochloric acid and enzymes break the food down while the stomach muscles act as a grinder, mechanically breaking less manageable chunks of food into smaller pieces. Finally, the stomach sterilizes bacteria before the food continues through the GI tract. At this point, the food is a somewhat fluid substance known as *chyme.*

The Small Intestine

Once food has been reduced to chyme, it is ready to journey through the small intestine. The small intestine has three sections—the *duodenum,* the *jejunum,* and the *ileum.* Chyme passes into the first section, the duodenum, through the pyloric sphincter muscle, which keeps it from being regurgitated back into the stomach.

The duodenum has cells that secrete digestive enzymes, acids, hormones, water, mucus, and ions to process the chyme further. The hormones regulate the secretion of bile and pancreatic juice into the duodenum at midpoint, and the chyme is processed with a shaking motion that mixes it with the secretions to aid in the digestion and absorption of nutrients. The next section of the small intestine, the jejunum, has a lining that absorbs carbohydrates and proteins from the chyme. The final section of the small intestine, the ileum, absorbs water, fat, bile, and salt. The ileum meets the large intestine at the valve known as the *ileocecal valve.* It prevents the backflow of material into the small intestine.

The Large Intestine

The large intestine, sometimes called the *colon,* moves the remaining matter, which is waste, from the small intestine to final elimination. As the waste passes through the ascendant colon to the transverse colon, more water is absorbed, until the waste is fairly firm. The muscles of the colon contract to squeeze the waste along through it. The ability of the colon to move waste through is referred to as *motility.* When the waste comes to the sigmoid colon, the last section of the large intestine, which empties into the rectum, colonic motility slows until the waste is released past the rectum, by voluntary relaxation of the sphincter muscle.

How Problems Arise

Clearly, the process of digestion is intense and complex. The gastrointestinal tract does an incredible amount of work digesting food, absorbing nutrients, and removing waste. In our world of fast food and hefty meals eaten on the run, the system frequently finds itself overtaxed—racing to keep up with increasing appetites and overburdened schedules. What happens when we give our GI tract more than it can handle?

Gas

Excess gas in the intestinal tract can produce a variety of unpleasant symptoms—oral release through burping and belching; rectal release of flatulence; cramping, and stomach distension from gas trapped in the tract.

The primary cause of excess gas is swallowed air. Air can be swallowed when eating too fast or gulping large chunks of food. People who breathe through their mouths may swallow air as they sleep. Nasal congestion and sinus problems may lead to gas trouble because they lead to mouth-breathing. Saliva is swallowed with air, so excess saliva production may cause gas problems, as may an extremely dry mouth, which prompts saliva secretion. Smoking and gum chewing both increase the amount of air swallowed, as do excessive yawning and sighing. Swallowing too much air is not, however, entirely caused by these physical actions. Significantly for the IBS sufferer, nerves and chronic anxiety regularly result in constant, and unconscious, ingestion of air.

A second source of gas is digestion of certain foods—those high in an undigestible carbohydrate, such as beans. The sugars in these foods draw bacteria into the large intestine. As the bacteria attack these sugars, hydrogen, carbon dioxide, and, on occasion, methane are released. The resulting flatulence, while unpleasant and embarrassing, rarely indicates a serious problem. It can generally be greatly improved by addressing both diet and poor dining habits, such as eating too fast or while on the run. For the IBS sufferer, at least temporary elimination of high-starch foods may offer noticeable relief and make it easier to track other triggers of the syndrome.

Cramping and Spasms

Gas trapped in the gastrointestinal system can be a cause of extreme cramping, which is also associated with a change in waste motility (constipation or diarrhea). Like flatulence, these cramps are frequently related to diet and can be caused by many things, from undercooked or spoiled food to lactose intolerance by a person. Regular cramping after meals is a common symptom of IBS.

Diarrhea

Diarrhea, the regular passage of soft and watery GI waste, occurs when waste moves more rapidly than is normal through the colon (in other words, when motility is increased). Two categories are generally recognized: acute, a condition with a rapid onset and a short, but severe, course of symptoms; and chronic, a lingering or ongoing condition. Acute diarrhea is prompted by viruses, bacteria, or parasites. Chronic diarrhea can result from a number of conditions that vary greatly in severity, from bothersome dietary responses such as lactose intolerance to life-threatening cancer of the bowel. Severe diarrhea itself can be life threatening.

Both acute and chronic instances of diarrhea may be linked to IBS. Studies have linked cases of acute bacterial and parasitic diarrhea to later ongoing problems with IBS. Chronic conditions that cause diarrhea, such as the inability to absorb fat, may not cause IBS, but treating them may nonetheless alleviate IBS symptoms. Perhaps most relevant to the IBS sufferer is the well-documented occurrence of nervous diarrhea, a condition in which tension, nerves, or depression increases waste motility.

Constipation

Constipation doesn't mean the same thing to everyone. Some people are used to having a bowel movement daily and find themselves uncomfortable if they go two or three days without one. Others normally have bowel movements no more than two or three times a week. Still others consider constipation to mean only that a bowel movement is difficult because of hardened stools, accompanied by cramping or rectal discomfort. Dietary patterns, such as the amounts of fiber and water ingested regularly, commonly affect the number of bowel movements a person usually experiences. Lack of exercise, a sudden change of diet (when traveling, for example), and not regularly responding to the immediate urge to defecate are some common, and benign, causes of constipation. More serious causes include rectal damage, colon cancer, Crohn's disease (an inflammatory disease of the ileum); and neuro-logical disorders such as cerebral palsy and multiple scle-rosis. Constipation may also occur in reaction to surgical procedures, drugs such as codeine, or fluid depletion. Un-like chronic diarrhea, constipation is not dangerous. For the IBS sufferer, diet and exercise changes are the best way to address the discomfort of constipation.

IBS Distress and the Mind/Body Connection

We owe a tremendous amount of our current understand-ing of how the stomach works to a pioneering army sur-geon named William Beaumont (1785–1853). After years of treating soldiers in the most brutal of conditions, Dr. Beaumont was stationed at Fort Mackinac on Lake Mich-igan near the Canadian border. There he met eighteen-year-old Alexis St. Martin, a voyageur, who collected furs from trappers and transported them via canoe to be sold. St. Martin suffered a severe musket injury to his upper abdomen, and Beaumont treated the wound, which he de-scribed as "more than the size of the palm of a man's hand," but he had little hope that the youth would survive. Survive he did, but the wound in his stomach never com-pletely healed. In the first years of his recovery, St. Martin stayed on to work as a handyman for Dr. Beaumont, and eventually he participated in the doctor's experiments. Be-cause St. Martin's stomach was partially exposed, with a hole into it, Beaumont was able to insert small pieces of food, attached to a string, through the hole and then re-move them after some hours to track the process of digestion. He could also directly observe the increase of gastric juice production during periods of stress or fear. Dr. Beaumont was the first to prove the mind/gut connection conclusively—that stomach problems as a result of stress were not simply in the sufferer's head but rather a physiologic response to increased production of gastric juice. Beaumont published a remarkable book, *Experiments and Observations on the Gastric Juice and the Physiology of Digestion,* which provides the basis for much of our understanding of stomach function. As for St. Martin, he eventually separated from Beaumont and, remarkably, lived to be eighty and father twenty children.

The mind/gut connection is vital to understanding IBS and offering useful and compassionate care for the IBS sufferer. The more IBS symptoms are understood as real physical reactions that are frequently triggered by psychological factors, rather than symptoms solely in the sufferer's mind, the more quickly and accurately the syndrome can be diagnosed and addressed. Equally important to a diagnosis is an understanding of what IBS is not or, more specifically, ruling out conditions that may have similar symptoms but are vastly different in their causes, severity, and treatment.

Differentiating Other Stomach Disorders

It is important to understand the similarities and differences between IBS and a number of other stomach disorders that may have symptoms in common. If you are experiencing any discomfort or troubling symptoms, *see a doctor immediately.* Under no circumstances should you attempt a self-diagnosis. That said, it is important to understand what IBS is not.

Inflammatory Bowel Disorder (IBD) is probably most often confused with IBS. Although the two may sound similar, they are very different. IBD is a far more serious, indeed sometimes life-threatening, disease that manifests in two forms—Crohn's disease and ulcerative colitis. Both of these conditions involve inflammation of the gastrointestinal tract and a thickening of the intestinal wall, in which deep ulcers may form. Both IBD diseases tend to arise during a person's late teens or early twenties, although they can strike at any time. With Crohn's disease, inflammation may occur anywhere from the mouth to the rectum; ulcerative colitis occurs in the colon (large intestine) and rectum. Symptoms of both include abdominal pain, fever, diarrhea, loss of appetite, weight loss, growth of an abdominal mass, and gastric bleeding. Bloody stools and rectal bleeding are more commonly found with ulcerative colitis than with Crohn's. Antibiotics, dietary adjustment, and, in the extreme, surgery, including colectomy (removal of all or part of the colon), may be used in the treatment of IBD. Colectomy may provide a cure for ulcerative colitis but not for Crohn's disease, although Crohn's disease sufferers may find their condition improved after surgery.

Colon cancer may occur in one out of twenty members of the population who have no known risk factors for the disease. For those who have suffered ulcerative colitis for more than ten years, the odds of developing cancer are thirty-two times higher than for the general population.

Any new and unusual symptoms that might indicate colon cancer should be addressed immediately. Examples include

- Unprovoked changes in bowel habits or stool consistency (in other words, changes that are not a reaction to changes in diet, changes in lifestyle, or illness)
- Bloody stools
- Persistent abdominal pain
- Difficulty in swallowing
- Consistent fullness after eating just a few bites

It's important to have an annual physical. If you are in a high-risk group, you may want to undergo annual or semiannual cancer screening for your own peace of mind, Should you detect an abnormality or disquieting symptoms at any time, see a doctor to greatly improve your chances for a full recovery.

Diverticulitis is an inflammation of an abnormal pouch (a *diverticulum;* the plural is *diverticula*) in the intestinal wall, usually in the large intestine (colon). Diverticula are about the size of a pea and form as a result of weakening in the lining of the intestine or simply as a result of aging, They occur with increasing frequency after age forty. Diverticula may exist in the intestinal lining without causing any symptoms; only when they are inflamed does a problem occur. Symptoms of diverticulitis include fever, elevated white blood cell count, and abdominal pain. If you have these symptoms, see a doctor immediately. If the diverticula become infected, the condition can be life threatening.

Diagnostic Criteria for IBS

Once doctors rule out a more serious illness, they apply two primary sets of criteria for identifying IBS: the Manning and the Rome criteria.

The Manning criteria have been in use since they were developed in the 1970s by a team of English researchers led by Dr. Manning. They establish an IBS diagnosis based on abdominal pain occurring more than six times in the previous year in combination with the following:

- Visible abdominal swelling
- Relief of stomach pain as a result of bowel movement
- Increased bowel movements with the onset of stomach pain
- Loose stools accompanying stomach pain
- Passage of mucus from the rectum
- Feeling that the bowel has not been completely evacuated after bowel movement

The more of these symptoms present, the greater the likelihood of an IBS diagnosis.

The Rome criteria were developed more recently for IBS diagnosis by a team of researchers in Rome. They establish an IBS diagnosis based on

1. At least three months of chronic or recurrent symptoms of abdominal pain or discomfort, generally in the lower abdomen, that is

+ Relieved by a bowel movement
+ Associated with a change in the frequency of bowel movements, whether an increase or a decrease
+ Associated with a change in stool consistency (either softer or harder)

2. Two or more of the following symptoms occurring every few days:

+ Altered stool frequency (more than three bowel movements a day or fewer than three in a week).
+ Altered stool form (hard or watery)
+ Altered stool passage (straining or difficulty during stool passage; urgency—the sudden need to rush to the bathroom for a bowel movement; or feeling that the bowel hasn't completed emptied after a bowel movement)
+ Passage of mucus (white matter) during a bowel movement
+ Bloating or a feeling of abdominal distension or fullness

Although you should never attempt self-diagnosis, knowledge of these criteria can help you talk candidly and clearly to your doctor. This will help the physician clearly identify the source of your gastric problems and begin the work of helping you to live better with IBS.

CHAPTER TWO

The Connection Between Body and Mind

For many years IBS sufferers were dismissed by physicians who asserted that their problems were "all in their minds." Fortunately, most doctors now know better, and people afflicted with IBS no longer have to be burdened by the trauma of enduring pain while being told that it's imaginary. Those misinformed practitioners did have one thing right—there is a connection between the mind and the GI tract. The fact is, the brain isn't creating or imagining the digestive troubles of the IBS sufferer, but it is involved in triggering them. There are two mental states most commonly associated with irritation in the GI tract: stress and depression.

Stress

All of us at one time or another have experienced the common symptoms that stress produces in our digestive system: "butterflies" in the stomach, cramping, the sudden need to go to the bathroom, nausea, and (in extreme cases) vomiting. IBS patients experience these symptoms of stress on a regular basis with daily stressors causing the most extreme of these physical reactions.

Stress, as defined by the *American Heritage Dictionary,* is "a state of extreme difficulty, pressure, or strain." Stress may be caused by external forces (from a lengthy traffic jam to an ailing loved one) or by internal forces (pressures we place upon ourselves). Whether it's the self-imposed deadline to make a million by the age of thirty, or the determination to maintain a perfectly clean house despite having two toddlers and a dog, many of us put undue stress on ourselves, which can have unfortunate physical consequences.

Hans Selye's Concept of Stress

What constitutes stress is highly personal and subjective. For instance, for someone who loves thrill rides, a roller coaster is an exciting treat. However, for someone who fears heights, just considering the long ride up to the first drop can make the stomach clench and the palms perspire. Hans Selye, who first developed the concept of stress and detailed it in his book *Stress of Life* (written in the 1930s), put it quite succinctly: "It is not what happens to you that matters, but how you take it." So stress is as much about the person undergoing the experience as it is about the experience itself, perhaps more.

Selye (1907–1982), a native of Vienna, published the first scientific paper to identify and define stress in 1936. He went beyond the popular notions of his day that healing involved identifying first the disease and then its specific remedy. He considered a broader view, that there was a "syndrome of just being sick." That notion, first known as "the general adaptation syndrome" and later as "the strain syndrome," was that strain, or stress, is a significant factor in the development of all types of disease. Selye believed that stress played a role in a variety of illnesses, ranging from mental disorders to high blood pressure and gastric ulcers, and that the similar symptoms experienced by patients with very different diseases were a result of the body's attempt to deal with the stress of being ill.

More than any researcher of his day or after, Selye clearly demonstrated and documented (in over fifteen hundred papers and thirty books) the role that our ability, or inability, to cope with stresses big and small plays in our health and well-being throughout our lives. We can also thank him for the increasingly popular and important focus on wellness, not as simply the absence of sickness but rather as a proactive and protective approach to caring for ourselves, body and mind.

Types of Stress

The gastrointestinal tract is particularly sensitive to stress and strain. It has sometimes been called "the second brain" because it contains so many nerve endings and its activities involve hormones and neurotransmitters (chemical substances in the body that transmit nerve impulses between neurons and cells). It is no coincidence that sadness may lead to loss of appetite, fear or nervousness to an urgent need to defecate. The "gut reaction" is very real. Let us consider in more detail the primary sources of the stress that causes these problems.

Survival stress is generated by a crisis situation, one that puts you in danger of immediate harm—physical or psychic. It could be provoked by an armed attacker or by the tantrum of an abusive boss. In reaction, the body releases adrenaline and prepares to fight or to flee. The average person does not regularly experience survival stress, although a battered wife or a resident of a violent and poverty-stricken neighborhood may unfortunately be familiar with it.

Internally generated stress is stress we create for ourselves. A worrier may fret constantly about things over which she has no control, anticipating worst-case scenarios in the future, such as "what if my computer crashes while I'm finishing my report," or "what if nobody shows up at my dinner." Living the event over and over in her mind, her anticipation creates more problems than the actual event ever could. A tense Type A person approaches life with the idea that everything must be under his control. The smallest problem gets blown up to major proportions. This is what makes the irate, red-faced restaurant patron shriek at the waiter because he has waited five minutes longer than anticipated for his lunch. The "stress junkie" lives in a catastrophe of her own making—bills always paid a day late, a long history of friends and lovers who "take advantage" of her, a series of jobs lost because of "bad bosses" or "impossible assignments." For her, the calm, ordered life is not worth living, although she would deny that she feels that way.

Environmental and job stress can arise because of a noisy neighbor, an inattentive landlord, a house in need of repair, a troublesome co-worker, an office short of staff. Some causes of this stress may be things you can change for the better; some you might learn to cope better with; and in some cases, you might have to abandon the situation altogether.

Fatigue and overwork cause stresses that build up over time. They may arise from deadlines that are self-imposed or imposed by others or by circumstance. Chronic fatigue and overwork generally result from two factors: an inability to manage time effectively and an inability to say no. These inabilities may be driven by the self-important belief that not only can you do it all but you can also do it better than anyone else; conversely they may arise from the self-deriding belief that people will like you only if you do their bidding. In either case, the long-term health effects can be seriously debilitating.

Stress Symptoms

To determine if you are under stress, consider whether you have these symptoms:

Physical Symptoms of Short-Term Stress
- Increased heart rate
- Sweating
- Cool skin
- Cold hands and feet
- Nausea
- "Butterflies in the stomach"
- Rapid breathing
- Muscle tensing
- Dry mouth
- A need to urinate
- Diarrhea

Physical Symptoms of Long-Term Stress

- Change in appetite
- Frequent colds
- Disorders such as asthma, back pain, digestive problems, headaches, skin eruptions
- Sexual disorders
- Aches and pains
- Feelings of intense and long-term fatigue

Psychological Symptoms of Short- or Long-Term Stress

- Worry and anxiety
- Confusion and inability to concentrate
- Feeling ill
- Feeling overwhelmed or out of control
- Mood changes, shifting between depression, frustration, hostility, helplessness, impatience, irritability, and restlessness
- Increasing lethargy
- Trouble sleeping
- Increased consumption of alcohol or cigarettes
- Change in eating habits—eating less or more or a drastic change in diet, such as constant and unusual consumption of junk food
- Reduced desire for sex
- Increased dependence on, and desire for, medication

IBS and Sensitivity to Stress

If several of the symptoms in any or all these categories describe you, you are likely suffering from excessive stress. If you believe you are also suffering from IBS, and believe there is a link between these stressors and your physical discomfort, you are doubtless correct. Whatever the stress, studies have shown that IBS sufferers have a lower tolerance for it, and a greater and more uncomfortable reaction to it, than does the general public.

Dr. Douglas Drossman, a gastroenterologist and co-director of the University of North Carolina Functional Gastrointestinal Disorder Center in Chapel Hill, reports that the bowels of people with IBS seem to react excessively in certain situations. "Anything that can affect the bowel in general will affect it more in people with IBS. It could be stress, diet, or activity." IBS patients need to discern what stressors trigger the symptoms, so that they can deal with them, as we will discuss in chapter seven.

Stress Symptoms as a Cause of Stress

An oddity about the mind/body connection and stress is worth noting. If you experience certain physical symptoms that are usually associated with stress, even if they are not in this instance caused by stress, they may actually induce stress in you. To explain this, consider caffeine. Suppose you've had one too many cups at breakfast, as many of us do. Not giving it a second thought, you go on about your day. Suddenly, you find your heart pounding, your thoughts wandering, your palms sweating. You have a momentary panic—what is happening? You become emotionally stressed because you feel physically stressed. The symptoms of panic create panic. The solution to this problem is awareness.

It is important to remember that physical problems can generate psychological reactions this way, when you're dealing with IBS and both stress and depression.

As gastroenterologist Joseph Sweeting at Columbia-Presbyterian Medical Center in New York City explains it, "There is no reason yet to conclude that psychological problems give rise to IBS. It's just as likely that IBS causes psychological problems."

Depression

IBS patients frequently experience depression, but the question of which came first, the symptom or the syndrome, is not definitively answered.

Cause or Effect of IBS?

The likelihood is that depression is more often a result of IBS than vice versa. It makes sense. Isolation is a major factor in depression, and increased isolation is often a result of IBS. Feeling embarrassed by their IBS symptoms, many sufferers turn down invitations to see family and friends rather than explain why they can no longer eat Aunt Linda's famous creamed spinach or why they've made five trips to the bathroom during dinner.

Depression can result from a feeling of hopelessness, and hopelessness can result from an IBS diagnosis, whether the physician is well informed about the condition or not. IBS sufferers who see a practitioner unfamiliar with the disease may be told it's all in their head, but they know it isn't. As a result, they feel relegated to a lifetime of pain and discomfort. They are also likely to feel frustrated and embarrassed by the doctor's dismissal of their complaint. IBS sufferers who go to a knowledgeable practitioner may be properly diagnosed, but the physician may offer no definitive course of treatment or prognosis for improvement. Who could help but be depressed when faced with the prospect of a lifetime of feeling uncomfortable and ill?

Other common causes of depression include

- The loss of a friend or relative
- A major disappointment at home or at work
- Prolonged or chronic illness
- Prescription drugs such as tranquilizers, high blood pressure medicine, steroids, codeine, and indomethacin
- Alcohol intoxication
- Alcohol withdrawal
- Drug intoxication
- Drug withdrawal

Distinguishing Depression from Other Feelings

Depression should not be confused with a passing feeling of sadness or the blues, although those feelings may be a part of depression. While there are varying degrees of depression, it occurs over a period of time and involves specific symptoms. To ascertain whether you're suffering from depression, consider the following:

- Do you regularly feel sad or blue?
- Do you no longer enjoy activities you once found pleasurable?
- Do you have a greatly diminished or nonexistent sex drive?
- Do you have difficulty doing things that used to be easy for you to do?
- Are you restless?

- Do you regularly feel fatigue?
- Have you experienced changes in sleeping patterns, dietary intake, or weight?
- Are you unable to make decisions?
- Do you feel worthless? Guilty? Pessimistic?
- Do you have thoughts of death or suicide?
- Are you experiencing a loss of concentration and/or diminished memory?

If you have five or more of these symptoms, you should consult a physician or therapist for a solid diagnosis and recommendation.

Types of Depression

There are three primary types of depression: major depression, dysthymia, and manic-depressive illness (now known as bipolar disorder).

A diagnosis of *major depression* is generally arrived at if most, or all, of the symptoms listed above are present for at least two weeks (and often longer). Major depression may strike only once or may recur several times in a person's life.

A diagnosis of *dysthymia* is arrived at if the sufferer has experienced the symptoms of major depression for a minimum of two years, but in a milder form than is manifested with major depression. Patients who suffer from dysthymia may periodically escalate into a major depression.

Manic-depressive illness is far less common than the other forms of depression. Sufferers experience a high and low cycle of behavior and mood swings, with depression in the lows and euphoria, irritable excitement, or manic behavior in the highs. Manic-depressive illness is a serious condition usually requiring long-term drug therapy in addition to psychological therapy.

Symptoms of mania include

- Abnormally elevated mood
- Irritability
- Severe insomnia
- Grandiose notions
- Increased talking
- Increasingly rapid thoughts
- Increased activity, including sex
- Noticeable increase in energy
- Risky behavior and regular use of poor judgment
- Inappropriate social behavior

When people exhibit the symptoms of major depression as a result of a substantial trauma, such as the death of a loved one, a divorce, or a business failure, but the symptoms are not severe enough to be considered a major depression, they are said to be suffering from *reactive depression.*

Many IBS patients suffer from major depression or dysthymia and can greatly benefit, both mentally and physically, from therapeutic intervention.

Therapy for Depression

Studies reported in the *Tufts University Health and Nutrition Letter* (September 1997) have shown that certain methods used to relieve mental strain also have physical benefits for IBS sufferers. Edward Blanchard, Ph.D., a clinical psychologist and researcher, has been considering psychological treatments for IBS since 1983. The public, however, has only recently begun to learn about the positive improvement in IBS symptoms that can result from these therapies. Dr. Blanchard lists three treatments that have so far been successful in treating some patients: brief psychodynamic therapy, cognitive behavioral therapy, and hypnosis.

Brief psychodynamic therapy is one-on-one treatment with a psychiatrist (M.D.) or psychologist (Ph.D.) over a brief period, typically once a week for two or three months. The sessions are used to detect possible unconscious triggers of IBS and to help patients become aware of what stressors may be causing their problem. The Tufts letter offers the example of a patient who may resent the way another person treats her but buries those feelings so that she is not aware of them. By internalizing the resentment, the patient causes herself emotional stress, and that triggers bowel symptoms.

Not only can brief therapy help reveal the truth of her resentments, but it can also offer solutions for dealing more constructively with her feelings. Once she stops internalizing her upset, her upset stomach is relieved as well. Although researchers can't offer a definitive explanation of why this therapy works, Dr. Blanchard reports that IBS patients who have undergone it subsequently report less pain and fewer bowel disturbances.

Cognitive behavioral therapy is also conducted by a psychiatrist or psychologist, but it can be done either solo or in groups. Cognitive therapy addresses the phenomenon of the patient sending himself conscious negative messages, perhaps holding himself more accountable than warranted when something goes wrong, imagining things to be worse than they genuinely are, or worrying about things that may or may not occur in the future.

In therapy, the patient is instructed to keep a record of his symptoms. Next, the therapy addresses the cause and effect between the negative messages he sends himself and the pain in his gut. The patient is then asked to closely examine his own life—where there is stress and where he himself contributes to that stress.

In the example offered, a patient might experience stress because of a work deadline. His first response is to say to himself, "I can't do it." That becomes "My boss thinks I'm a loser," then the thought "I'm going to lose my job," and so on, in a downward spiral of thought that is known as *catastrophizing*.

Once the patient has learned how he is contributing to and increasing his own stress, he then learns a new way to talk to himself. He is encouraged to address his problems more realistically, asking himself, for instance, "If I can't meet my deadline, does it really make me completely incompetent?" Over time, he can reverse the trend of escalating difficult situations and can learn to cope in a calm and positive way.

Although Dr. Blanchard cannot ascertain exactly why, his research has shown a significant reduction in IBS symptoms for patients undergoing cognitive therapy.

The third therapy that has shown promise, *hypnosis,* is discussed in detail in chapter seven.

Other current research on the mind/gut connection focuses on the *enteric nervous system,* a system of nerve cells located throughout the digestive tract. This complex neural network both talks to the brain and functions independently of it. Michael Gershon, a biologist at Columbia-Presbyterian Medical Center in New York, puts it this way: "The gut's not just a passive tube. It has a mind of its own, and we're just beginning to understand how that mind works." Dr. Gershon's research has revealed that brain chemicals called *neurotransmitters* have a direct effect on digestion. His research focuses on *serotonin,* the neurotransmitter that plays a role in psychological well-being, and he believes it may provide the key to improved treatment of IBS. His studies involve adjusting the amount of serotonin available to cells in the digestive tract to see how this speeds or slows the digestive process, altering irritability of the gut.

The mind/gut connection is clear. In later chapters we'll address ways to identify stressors in your own life and offer some positive coping methods.

CHAPTER THREE

The Female Factor

Irritable bowel syndrome is diagnosed in women twice as often as it is in men. In the largest and most comprehensive study done on the syndrome "IBS in American Women" (1999, funded by Glaxo Pharmaceuticals), nearly three thousand people—including women with and without IBS, physicians, pharmacists, and nurses—were interviewed in depth by phone, and their responses revealed some fascinating facts.

Nearly 40 percent of women suffering from IBS reported abdominal pain that they described as intolerable. Even those women whose pain was not that intense stated that IBS symptoms forced them to miss work, limit travel, or avoid going out socially. Despite that, doctors who treated IBS rated the pain as significantly less severe than their patients did. Further, many stated that, although IBS may be distressing, it is not a serious medical condition.

Doctors' Attitudes

Why do doctors so often dismiss functional disorders such as IBS? In the *Journal of Addiction and Mental Health* (May/June 2000), Dr. Brenda Toner, head of both the Women's Mental Health Research Section at the Centre for Addiction and Mental Health and the Women's Mental Health Program at the University of Toronto, where she is an associate professor of psychiatry, believes that "It comes from our need [in Western society] to elevate the organic, while still viewing any psychological attributes of illness as pejorative or shameful or somehow the individual's fault." In other words, if a specific physical cause for a problem hasn't been identified, physicians greatly diminish their opinion of its legitimacy and impact and often convey a sense that the patient is either imagining or somehow to blame for the symptoms.

This lack of understanding of, and effective treatment for, IBS affects not only patients but also their families and society as a whole. Economically IBS has a very real impact—women with IBS miss work two to three times as often as women without it. One in four has to allow extra commute time, or is late to work, because of the condition. The relationships of friends and family with the IBS patient may be adversely affected by the sufferer's need to limit her activities—because of either discomfort or embarrassment. Two out of three women with active IBS are concerned about, and plan schedules and activities around, the location of restrooms.

Many women who suffer from IBS wonder whether their illness isn't taken as seriously as it should be precisely because they are women. There is, after all, a long tradition in Western medicine of dismissing the "hysterical female." Whatever the reason for doctors' attitudes toward IBS, women are now speaking out and making a difference for those suffering from the condition. In 1991, Nancy Norton set up the International Foundation for Functional Gastrointestinal Disorders, based in Milwaukee, Wisconsin, because she found so little support, education, and information available during her own struggles with IBS. In the *Journal of Addiction and Mental Health* (May/June 2000), Norton states: "Historically, patients with a diagnosis of IBS have been treated as if their symptoms are psychosomatic [and therefore] illegitimate." The good news is, she sees a change. "I think we're beginning to see the stigma . . . go away."

Dr. Lin Chang, co-director of the UCLA Neurocentric Disease Center and technical director for the 1999 study "IBS in American Women," believes that women patients may indeed be treated differently. In an interview for the Web site Intellihealth, Dr. Chang stated, "A lot of women IBS patients, and women patients in general, feel that there is some difference in the way a doctor treats a male vs. a female patient." However, she believes that a lack of knowledge, more than the gender gap, results in incorrect diagnosis and improper treatment of IBS sufferers by doctors.

The problem of uninformed doctors is clearly outlined in "IBS and American Women." Nearly 80 percent of the doctors surveyed did not follow the published and established criteria for an IBS diagnosis. Fewer than 20 percent said they were "somewhat familiar" with the criteria. And 87 percent said that their profession, as a whole, needs to be better educated about IBS.

To take control of this condition and their lives, women have to learn as much as possible about IBS, particularly those factors and triggers that are primarily identified with female sufferers: sexual and emotional abuse, the menstrual cycle, and the common female habit of trying to be all things to all people, which has been called "the disease to please."

IBS and Childhood Sexual Abuse

Although this section specifically addresses women's experiences of childhood sexual abuse and a later diagnosis of IBS, I am well aware that the issues discussed here affect many men as well. However, the stigma of reporting both abuse and IBS is much greater for men—although women certainly are stigmatized also—and therefore women are far more likely to report these experiences. The available data thus focus on females, and those data are far from clear-cut.

Recent studies have shown that as many as 50 percent of women diagnosed with IBS have been victims of physical, sexual, or emotional abuse. Despite that, the cause-and-effect relationship between childhood abuse and an IBS diagnosis has not been well established. A history of sexual abuse has also been identified as a contributing factor in other bowel syndromes and chronic pelvic pain. And emotional and physical abuse during childhood have been associated with IBS.

A few associations between IBS and abuse other than direct cause and effect are possible. Primary among them is the finding that those who suffered an abusive childhood continue to suffer into adulthood, generally experiencing more stress and unhappiness than those who had a positive upbringing. In addition to painful memories, these adults also continue to suffer from the lack of a family support system—they may not have anyone to turn to when things get rough, or they may be afraid or unable to ask for help even if it is available. Finally, the very coping mechanisms of denial and repression that allowed them to live through the abuse, combined with the self-loathing and guilt experienced by many abuse survivors, often lead to an extreme internalization of problems and fears. As we discussed in chapter two, internalized emotions—along with stress—frequently lead to a "gut reaction," which may trigger IBS.

Another possible relationship between childhood abuse and IBS is simply that the physical and mental problems that abuse survivors experience as a result of their trauma make them more likely than the general population to seek medical attention, for either physical or emotional reasons. Dealing with one problem may lead to a diagnosis of the other.

Whether abuse victims are actually more likely to experience IBS, or just more likely to come forward with their symptoms and be diagnosed, they are likely to experience more severe symptoms of the syndrome because the ongoing stress of their lives makes them more susceptible to pain. Interestingly, IBS is not the only functional disorder that has been linked to past sexual abuse. Fibromyalgia, a chronic condition of muscle and skeletal pain and chronic fatigue, which we'll discuss in more detail in chapter four, is also a common condition among abuse victims. In this disorder, like IBS, the primary impact of a history of abuse is an increased severity of symptoms.

A 1999 study at the University of Toronto examined the issue of emotional abuse and IBS. The researchers questioned twenty-five women about experiences of emotional abuse that they defined as psychological mistreatment and nonphysical aggression. The study also tested subjects for two psychosocial factors that likely factor into IBS—self-silencing and self-blame.

Self-silencing is the attempt to keep various relationships secure and intact by refraining from expressing actions, feelings, and thoughts that may upset or anger the other people in those relationships. Practiced over the long term, self-silencing can lead to complete loss of your sense of self and self-worth. *Self-blame* is a tendency to constantly criticize yourself and take the blame for everything that may go wrong around you—at home, at work, and with friends.

The Toronto study, published in *Psychosomatic Medicine* (January/February 2000), found that participants with IBS scored significantly higher on all three factors—emotional abuse, self-blame, and self-silencing—than participants without IBS. Researchers believe that, yet again, the stress of these emotional burdens contributes to—and triggers—IBS.

While more research about the relationship between abuse and IBS needs to be done before cause and effect can be clearly established, one thing does seem certain—sexual or physical abuse is not a physical cause of IBS. Whatever physical harm is done to the child, and whatever other medical problems result, the abuse does not cause structural damage or alteration of the GI tract that would cause IBS. Rather, by creating an environment of stress and unhappiness, it contributes to the triggering of IBS symptoms.

The cognitive therapies discussed in chapter two and the stress management techniques discussed in chapter six can go a long way toward relieving IBS for survivors of abuse.

Effects of the Menstrual Cycle

Many women who do not suffer from IBS have abdominal problems when their period is due, but the number is much higher among IBS sufferers. Up to 50 percent of women with IBS report increased premenstrual syndrome (PMS) symptoms, and studies show that IBS patients experience increased gas and cramping at menstruation. Although many patients experienced increased diarrhea or constipation as well, those findings are not as consistently present. Many other medical conditions, including migraine, asthma, and epilepsy, are exacerbated by the menstrual cycle.

It is important to keep a record of your symptoms to fully understand how your period affects your experiences with IBS. IBS symptoms are frequently exacerbated during the postovulatory and premenstrual phases of the cycle, likely as a result of hormonal changes. During the ovulatory phase, progesterone is dominant, and many women report constipation during this time. Progesterone has well-documented effects on the gastrointestinal tract, including delaying gastric elimination. Slower transit of waste matter through the GI tract has also been documented during this phase of the menstrual cycle.

The most abrupt change in bowel habits occurs at the start of the menstrual flow. At this point, progesterone levels fall, which triggers an increase in bowel activity in some women. At the same time, levels of prostaglandin E2 and F2 alpha—hormones shown to be powerful stimulants of colonic contraction—rise. IBS patients, whose colons are generally hyperresponsive and hypersensitive to a number of stimuli, may have an extreme colonic response to the release of prostaglandins during menstruation.

Some women have had success in treating bowel disorders with ovarian suppression therapies and complete elimination of the menstrual cycle; however, the expense and adverse side effects associated with these treatments in the long term generally preclude their prolonged use. If bowel problems associated with menstruation are extraordinarily debilitating, and ovarian suppression has offered some relief, in rare instances ovariectomy and low-dose estrogen replacement may have a therapeutic role.

Interestingly, a small study suggests that women whose IBS symptoms are closely tied to the menstrual cycle may be less likely to seek medical attention than women with other IBS triggers. A study of three groups of women—those diagnosed with IBS; those who had not been diagnosed but had all the symptoms of IBS; and those who had no IBS symptoms—revealed that those who experienced IBS with menstruation simply considered it a normal, if uncomfortable, symptom of their menstrual cycle and, as a result, did not seek help for the condition.

In general, the best approach to minimizing the problems of IBS and periods is to track your symptoms and avoid stress and food triggers during the most problematic times of your cycle (see chapters five and six).

The Disease to Please

There is no greater culprit in IBS than stress. And one of the major causes of stress in women is a condition that became part of the popular lexicon after being featured on the *Oprah Winfrey Show:* the disease to please.

Do you find it impossible to say no? Do you worry that others will no longer like you if you aren't always available to them? Is it important to you that everyone view you as kind, caring, and giving all the time? Does the thought of confronting or contradicting someone seem almost overwhelming? Are you frightened and upset by the notion that anyone is upset or angry with you? If these questions paint a picture that seems familiar, you may be suffering from the disease to please.

Putting everyone's needs and happiness before your own may seem to be the "good" thing to do, but the truth is that it can do real damage. Anxiety, stress, depression, irritability, headaches, sleeplessness, and GI problems—these are all common symptoms of the woman who's there for everyone but herself.

A contributor to this ever-growing syndrome is the fact that an increasing number of women are balancing work and home duties. Brought up to be agreeable and accommodating, with the notion that females are the primary family nurturers and caretakers, many women try to be ideal homemakers while working full-time jobs. These are the women who come home from work only to set about making the house spotless in-between runs to soccer practice and the supermarket. Of course, real nurturing can't occur on the run, and although the family situation may look good on the surface, many of the most important things in life—spontaneity, time to dream, the relaxed enjoyment of family and friends—are sacrificed to this constant activity.

Ironically, the disease to please may actually draw toxic people into a woman's life. Most healthy, balanced people want a reasonable give and take in a relationship and aren't comfortable with someone who is always putting herself last. Consequently, the pleaser may find herself disproportionately surrounded by takers: the friend who can talk about nothing but herself; the boss who dumps all the work on her and then takes the credit; the neighbor who regularly drops by for a minute and stays for two hours. The pleaser's inability to say no robs her of time with positive and productive friends and family.

If you're suffering from this syndrome, consider the many ways it can affect IBS. First, there is the stress of an overloaded schedule. Then there is the likelihood that you will internalize the frustration and resentment inherent in your attempt to be all things to all people. Third, when time is of the essence, diet inevitably suffers and exercise is placed on the back burner.

If learning to say no seems frightening, consider what *not* learning to say no could mean—a lifetime of poor health, strained relationships, unhappiness, and lack of satisfaction in day-to-day life.

A detailed approach to managing this syndrome and other stressors appears in chapter seven, but right now you can begin thinking about the realities of your daily life and the effects of trying to keep everyone happy. Ask yourself these questions:

- How are the good people in your life short-changed by the time you give the takers?
- How is your health affected by your schedule?
- How often do health problems literally force you to stop what you are doing, leaving you further behind and more overwhelmed than you already were?
- What do you believe will happen if you say no?
- What do you believe will happen if someone is angry with you?
- What do you believe will happen if someone doesn't like you?
- Do you regularly do things you have no desire to do to gain others' approval?
- Is it more important to you to be liked or to be respected?
- Which of your daily tasks, either at home or at work, could you easily give to others to alleviate your schedule?
- What would your days be like if you did what you really needed and wanted to, rather than what others feel you should do?

This chapter has outlined many triggers specific to women with IBS. The next chapter addresses chronic conditions that may trigger, or overlap, an IBS diagnosis. Like IBS, some of these conditions are disproportionately diagnosed in women.

CHAPTER FOUR

Disorders Commonly Linked with IBS

A s if dealing with IBS weren't enough, IBS sufferers commonly experience other functional disorders or, conversely, have functional disorders that trigger IBS. This chapter considers some of the chronic conditions most frequently linked with IBS and how they may trigger or exacerbate the condition. It also looks at three physical conditions —acute and bacterial gastroenteritis, food allergies, and alcohol dependency—that may trigger IBS.

Functional Disorders and IBS

Fibromyalgia

Fibromyalgia, like IBS, is a functional disorder, and patients with fibromyalgia are frequently diagnosed as also having IBS. Fibromyalgia is characterized by widespread pain in muscles, tendons, fibrous tissues, and other connective tissues. Muscle pain is widespread, but it does not lead to weakness. For fibromyalgia to be positively diagnosed, pain must be present in eleven of eighteen specific tender sites when they are pressed.

Fibromyalgia sufferers generally ache all over, experience stiffness when walking, and are fatigued. The condition often runs in families and can be triggered by injury, infection, stress, or sleep disturbance. Two previous theories of fibromyalgia—that it was an arthritic disorder and that it was psychosomatic—have not proved true. There is no solid evidence of inflammation, which would be necessary for a diagnosis of arthritis. As for the pain, fibromyalgia patients have shown four times the normal level of the primary neurotransmitter for pain (substance P) in their spinal fluid, indicating that the pain indeed is real.

Although the cause of fibromyalgia is not clear, studies have produced some plausible theories and solid data. Increasingly abnormality of deep sleep has been identified and researched as a likely contributor to fibromyalgia. Patients frequently report that not getting enough sleep, or even staying up later than usual, makes their symptoms worse the next day. Studies have shown abnormal brain wave forms in fibromyalgia patients during deep sleep. Volunteers who are free of fibromyalgia have had symptoms of the syndrome and tenderness induced by deprivation of deep sleep over a period of several days.

Fibromyalgia patients often have low levels of growth hormone, and growth hormone is produced almost exclusively during deep sleep. Growth hormone is important in maintaining the health of muscles and soft tissues. Exercise and good sleep can increase growth hormone production and improve the condition of fibromyalgia patients.

Fibromyalgia is associated with changes in the immune system similar to those that appear when a person is fighting a virus. However, no virus is present, and the condition is not contagious. Again, sleep disturbance may be the culprit, as loss of deep sleep has been shown to result in similar immune system changes.

The fibromyalgia patient can receive significant relief of symptoms from proactive changes in lifestyle. Like IBS, fibromyalgia does not get better with short-term treatment. It may be treated with the following:

- Medication, such as Elavil, Benadryl, or Xanax, to improve deep sleep.
- Establishment of regular patterns and ample amounts of sleep.
- Daily participation in a regimen of gentle exercise and stretching.
- Avoidance of stress and overexertion whenever possible.

Anything that disturbs sleep is to be avoided. Alcohol, caffeine, and other stimulants should not be ingested, particularly in the evening. Exercise should be done in the morning, because any exertion within three or four hours of bedtime can disrupt sleep. All these practices will likely reduce IBS symptoms as well.

Nonulcer Dyspepsia

Dyspepsia is recurrent or chronic pain in the upper abdomen. It may have a specific cause, such as an ulcer, cancer, or a disease of the liver, pancreas, or bile duct. *Nonulcer dyspepsia* is dyspepsia that appears as a functional disorder with no identifiable cause. Like IBS, nonulcer dyspepsia has a set of Rome criteria to establish the diagnosis. The criteria include at least three months of chronic or recurrent symptoms of pain or discomfort focused in the upper abdomen, with no known disease or disorder detected to account for the symptoms.

Dyspepsia is felt in the upper abdomen and should not be confused with chest pain or heartburn, although these conditions may occur simultaneously. If you experience chronic dyspepsia visit your doctor, because only through tests can the cause be determined and other ailments be ruled out. The doctor can determine whether your specific experience of dyspepsia is a functional disorder or a symptom of some graver problem.

There are no drug treatments for nonulcer dyspepsia, and there are drugs you should avoid if you have been diagnosed with it. Aspirin and nonsteroidal anti-inflammatories (NSAIDs) such as ibuprofen (Advil) can irritate and inflame the stomach. Avoid them in favor of pain relievers such as acetaminophen (Tylenol) that do not disrupt the stomach. Alcohol, tobacco, and caffeine are also irritants and should be avoided. Antacids do not relieve dyspepsia and may cause diarrhea, so they are best avoided when symptoms of IBS are also present. Interestingly, nonulcer dyspepsia is often relieved once the patient has a diagnosis confirming that the condition is not caused by a serious illness and will not itself create serious problems.

Although both IBS and dyspepsia involve pain in the upper abdomen, IBS is likely to be the diagnosis when pain is accompanied by diarrhea or constipation. While it's unpleasant to suffer both conditions, treatment strategies offer hope that the symptoms of both conditions can be relieved.

Globus Hystericus

Having a "lump in your throat" when no lump or other physical cause is present is known as *globus hystericus*. It is more common in women than in men and generally occurs during times of anxiety or stress. Globus hystericus is a *conversion syndrome*—that is, a syndrome of psychological stress that manifests in a physical way. It gets its name from the outdated notion that such a symptom is "hysterical"—all in the patient's head, instead of an actual physical condition that can be triggered in the mind.

The experience of globus hystericus, like all functional disorders, varies from person to person. If no physical cause is detected, some simply find it a mild annoyance while others may actually have difficulty eating and swallowing due to the sensation of a blocked throat. The condition may occur following problems in the GI tract or other stress-related conditions.

People suffering globus hystericus, like those with nonulcer dyspepsia, sometimes experience relief of anxiety and, as a result, of the symptomatic lump in the throat, simply from the reassurance that globus hystericus is not linked to any serious underlying cause. Treatment of the disorder involves a variety of stress reducers, including exercise and meditation. If the problem persists, a brief course of tranquilizers or anti-anxiety medication may be called for.

Physical Disorders That May Trigger IBS

While not the root cause of IBS, certain diagnosable diseases and conditions can exacerbate or trigger the syndrome.

Acute and Bacterial Gastroenteritis

It is not uncommon for IBS to manifest after a person has experienced a bout of acute gastroenteritis or infectious diarrhea. This is diarrhea resulting from ingestion of infected or contaminated water or food. Nausea, vomiting, and severe abdominal pain and diarrhea result from the body's efforts to get rid of the toxins. Once the episode ends, although patients are likely to feel exhausted and not well overall, they usually recover fully and fairly rapidly.

In a study detailed in *The Lancet* (January 20, 1996), seventy-five patients with acute gastroenteritis were given a series of psychometric tests soon after entering the hospital. Participants ranged in age from eighteen to eighty. Anyone who had previously exhibited or suffered symptoms of IBS was excluded, as were patients who took medications that might affect bowel habits. A detailed medical history was taken, recording the duration of the acute illness, the severity of the symptoms, and the use of antibiotics in treatment.

Patients completed questionnaires addressing depression, anxiety, personality traits, and physical symptoms, including insomnia, headaches, dizziness, shortness of breath, musculoskeletal pain, and backache. Any symptoms that had an organic basis were discounted. These tests were repeated at three months, and then at six.

Twenty-two of the seventy-five patients experienced symptoms of IBS following the acute illness, and six months later twenty of them still showed persistent symptoms. Those with IBS symptoms tested higher for anxiety, depression, and neurotic traits than the rest of the group, and their scores were unchanged at the three-month follow-up.

The study found that the intensity of the original gastric disturbance was not a factor in later development of IBS symptoms, although the length of the incident was—those with IBS had endured the longest bouts of acute diarrhea. More women than men went on to develop IBS.

The study concluded that the development of IBS was probably not a direct result of any structural changes resulting from the gastroenteritis but rather a psychological response. For patients with already high levels of stress and anxiety, the trauma of a gastrointestinal attack can be a psychological trigger for IBS. This underlines the importance of understanding and treating psychological factors when dealing with IBS.

Alcohol Abuse or Dependence

In a study reported in the *American Journal of Drug and Alcohol Abuse* (August 1998), thirty-one patients seeking treatment for drug and alcohol abuse were compared with an age- and sex-matched control group of forty patients seeking treatment from a general physician for other medical problems. Among the control group, 2.5 percent met the criteria for IBS. Among those with drug and alcohol issues, the number was an astonishing 41.9 percent.

Why so high a figure? Remember, first of all, that this small preliminary study doesn't offer definitive answers as much as it raises questions and considerations. What we do know is that alcohol is a stimulant, both to the appetite and to the digestive tract. This is where the notion of an aperitif—a small cocktail before dining—comes from. The word literally means a stimulant to the bowels. Unfortunately, the last thing an IBS sufferer needs is stimulation of the gastrointestinal tract, and alcohol may trigger abdominal pain, cramping, diarrhea, and heartburn.

Depression is also a trigger for IBS, and depression is also common among those suffering from alcohol or drug dependence. When an individual becomes dependent on alcohol or drugs, the stresses of daily life inevitably increase. Unpaid bills, tumultuous relationships, missed deadlines, and lost work are common when alcohol or drugs are abused. Again, stress is a common IBS trigger.

Some alcohol products may physically trigger IBS. Beer, in particular, may be a serious trigger, because it has a high yeast content and yeast is a common food trigger for IBS patients.

Alcohol or drug abuse and IBS have the potential to create a truly vicious circle. Alcohol triggers the symptoms of IBS, which can leave the sufferer feeling ill and depressed, isolated and hopeless. Those feelings frequently contribute to the desire to drink or take drugs. As alcoholism or drug abuse advances, the tendency to neglect diet—either eating poorly or not at all—increases. Exercise is generally abandoned. These all contribute to the problems of IBS.

If you suffer from alcoholism or believe you are overdependent on alcohol or drugs, and you suspect that you may also have IBS, it's important to consult a doctor for both conditions. Physical relief of your painful symptoms may motivate you to take better control of your life and health. Understanding how stress and depression can trigger both your digestive problems and the need for alcohol or drugs may help you better understand both conditions and offer the hope that you can, indeed, feel happy and healthy again—a hope that is vital to your recovery.

Food Allergies

Many people believe that they or their family members suffer from food allergies, but in fact only 2 to 8 percent of the population are truly allergic. For a true allergy to be present, the body must have an immune system response to the food in question. Peanuts and shellfish are two of the foods most commonly causing allergies, and both can cause severe reactions, even death, if the allergic person inadvertently consumes them.

True food allergies generally cause some or all of the following reactions:

- Itching
- Hives
- Eczema
- Irritated and itching eyes
- Tightening of the throat
- Wheezing

- Coughing
- Nausea and vomiting
- Diarrhea

True allergic food reactions almost always occur within thirty minutes of eating the offending item. The longer the time between ingestion and reaction to it, the more likely it is that the problem is an intolerance of or sensitivity to the offending item, rather than a genuine allergy.

If you have been diagnosed with a food allergy (see chapter five), it is important to exclude not only that food but also extracts of it from your diet. Peanut oil, for instance, is as harmful as the nut in its whole form.

If you think you may have food allergies, consider your reactions to the following:

- Milk and dairy products
- Chicken eggs
- Fish and shellfish such as shrimp or oysters
- Peanuts and other nuts, such as walnuts, that grow on trees
- Gluten, which is found in wheat, rye, barley, and some oats
- MSG (the food additive monosodium glutamate)
- Other food additives such as dyes and colorings

Fortunately, most negative reactions to food fall into the category of food intolerance, not allergy.

Food Intolerance

Food intolerance is determined much as IBS is—by symptoms rather than a physiologic reaction, or finding, that can be definitively diagnosed by a doctor.

Food intolerance suggests a reaction that builds over time. The occasional bit of cheese or bread may not cause a problem, for instance, but large amounts, or daily consumption, can lead to any, or all, of the gut reactions common to IBS sufferers. Keeping a food diary (a process outlined in chapter 5) is a good way to determine which foods you might have difficulty tolerating. If you think you may have a food intolerance, consider your reaction to the following:

Lactose, the sugar found in milk, is difficult for many people to digest. In fact lactose intolerance has become a well-known phenomenon, sparking lactose-free products and the creation of aids for lactose digestion. Lactose-rich foods include cows' milk and ice cream. Butter, margarine, and cheeses also contain lactose, although in lower concentrations.

Wheat and wheat products may cause intolerance reactions different from the allergic reaction caused by gluten. Wheat-sensitive people may experience a triggering of IBS symptoms after excessive consumption of bread, crackers, and pasta. Wheat restriction, rather than elimination, is the answer for them.

Fructose intolerance, while not as common as other intolerances, does affect some IBS sufferers. Dried fruits and fruit juices are frequently high in fructose. It is also a major component of corn syrup, which is used as a sweetener for syrups, jams, jellies, pastry glazes, cereals, and soft drinks. If you regularly experience a gut reaction to these products, read food labels carefully to discover if fructose is an ingredient.

Sorbitol is a nonabsorbable sugar commonly added to diet candies, breath mints, chewing gum, and medicines to make them more palatable. Although it may improve the taste of some food items, it unfortunately creates problems for a great many people, not just those with IBS. It should be avoided whenever possible, particularly if you suffer from cramps or diarrhea. It's important to read labels to discover whether the foods you eat contain sorbitol, and then see whether it creates problems for you.

PART TWO

How to Manage IBS: Treatments and Strategies

NOW THAT YOU HAVE TAKEN A LOOK at the symptoms and triggers of IBS, and disorders that may be related or linked to it, it's time for you to chart your personal experience of the syndrome and map your strategy to begin living far better with the condition.

First, if you believe you have IBS but have yet to be diagnosed by your physician, now is the time to do so. By going to your doctor with some understanding of IBS, you will be more able than many patients to articulate your problems and assist the physician in reaching a diagnosis. The doctor will

- Take a complete medical history
- Do a general, physical examination
- Take blood and stool samples
- Possibly order X rays or a bowel examination using a scope

Once any other cause has been eliminated, and you have been determined to exhibit symptoms established by either the Manning or the Rome criteria or both, a diagnosis of IBS is made. Then it's time to determine exactly how the syndrome affects you. To develop a clear picture of how IBS affects you personally, you need to answer several questions:

- When do you first remember experiencing symptoms of IBS?
- What daily food choices trigger your symptoms of IBS?
- What situations may lead to a bout of IBS?
- Which (if any) of the conditions that may trigger or overlap IBS do you suffer from?

To answer many of these questions, you need to keep two detailed diaries—one for diet and one for stressors. This may seem an unnecessary process, a task that you simply don't have the time or inclination to undertake. But I ask you to consider how much of your life is being taken up by IBS. If you realistically answer that question, it should be clear that you cannot afford *not* to take care of yourself.

Remember, relief from IBS is not an overnight remake. Nor is the program of keeping diaries and making changes so extensive that it will be hard to attempt, let alone sustain. Rather, this process is about small, manageable steps that will enable you to get a little better day by day while doing things that work within the context of both your lifestyle and your belief systems. You really can feel good again—and now you'll begin the journey to get there.

CHAPTER FIVE

Diet Strategies

W hat you eat and how and when you eat it affect all aspects of your health. You don't have to have IBS to know the discomfort that can result from gulping down a burger on the run or overloading your stomach with gas-producing vegetables and legumes. For the IBS sufferer, however, these problems are magnified. What might be a one-time incident of stomach upset for an individual free of IBS may be a chronic reaction for an IBS patient.

Keeping a Food Diary

The first thing to know is that food affects each sufferer differently. What may trigger symptoms in one won't trigger them in another. That's why it's vital to start the process of finding relief by keeping a detailed food diary. Two things are important to making this an honest, and therefore useful, record of your food triggers:

1. Record everything. All of us have a tendency to want to record our best selves—witness the dieter who, while honestly keeping a journal of her daily intake, may fail to note the half brownie nibbled after lunch or that after-dinner candy. Even though she's the only one who will read the record, she's loathe to record what she considers bad behavior.

2. Don't alter your behavior during the initial recording period. So much is discussed about which foods are good and which are bad that you may assume that a food will affect you and eliminate it during the tracking process. Don't. It's important to maintain your regular routine to get an honest picture of your food reactions. You may well be surprised by what does and doesn't trigger your IBS symptoms.

With those two rules well in hand, here's what you need to record in your food diary:

- Everything you eat and drink—not simply full meals, but also the half cup of coffee at mid-morning, the Snickers bar in the car, the two bites of a peanut butter sandwich absentmindedly nibbled while unpacking your child's un-eaten lunch. All these are important.

- How much you actually ate. For instance, "cheeseburger" doesn't really tell the story. Was it a Quarter Pounder or a Big Mac? Differences in the quantity of beef and the condiments used (ketchup or "secret sauce," for instance) may offer a clue about what triggers your IBS. Be sure to differentiate between what you were served and what you actually consumed. For instance, suppose you go out to lunch and order pot roast with mashed potatoes, gravy, and broccoli. But is that what you ate? We all know people who leave the vegetables untouched, or skip the gravy, or religiously save half the meal for dinner. Consider the salad: Was it iceberg lettuce with a full ladle of ranch dressing, or a variety of greens, carrots, and tomatoes with oil and vinegar? Did you leave the croutons piled on the side of your plate, or did you devour them and request bacon bits in addition?

→ How much you drank and whether food was involved. Did you have two cups of coffee with breakfast or on an empty stomach? Did you have one coke with lunch or were there several refills? How many glasses of water did you consume and when?

→ Under what circumstances you ate and drank. Did you have a sandwich standing alone over the kitchen sink or sitting down with family and friends? Did you gulp it down in two minutes or eat it slowly? Did you eat in a relaxed atmosphere or surrounded by the distractions of ringing phones or crying children?

→ What happened after you ate. Did you experience any abdominal pain? Cramps? Diarrhea? If so, how intense? Did you have gas, either belching or flatulence, or a feeling of bloat or excessive fullness? Did your abdomen become distended? How long after eating or drinking did these symptoms occur? How long did they last?

The best approach is probably to keep this diary in two ways. First, keep a small notebook with you at all times to jot down food and drink, circumstances, and any reactions. Then use this notebook to create a log at home that you fill in completely each night before bed.

A two-week diary should give you a clear picture of the food and eating habits that trigger your IBS. Women who believe their IBS symptoms may be linked to their menstrual periods may want to include the weeks immediately before and after their periods in their diaries to determine if hormonal changes affect food triggers.

Analyzing Your Diet Diary

When you review your diary, certain foods are likely to leap out as regularly being present before an IBS attack. They may be unexpected, or they may be quite common.

Common Trigger Foods

Let's look at some food groups that commonly trigger IBS and how those foods may affect the digestive tract.

Fats

Fats, such as butter, margarine, oil, peanut butter, mayonnaise, and salad dressing, along with fatty cuts of meat and fried foods, are common causes of digestive problems for those who suffer from IBS (and those who don't). The reason is that the hormonal system releases chemicals—

particularly cholecystokinin—to promote the digestive processing of the fat, but these chemicals also trigger abnormal movement and contractions in the colon.

Dairy Products

Problems that result from eating dairy products are generally a result of lactose intolerance—the inability to digest significant amounts of lactose, which is the predominant sugar found in milk. This inability is due to a shortage of the enzyme lactase, which is produced by the cells lining the small intestine. In high-fat dairy products, such as brie, hard cheeses, and ice cream, fat may also be a factor in the digestive difficulties.

High-Fiber Foods

Often people suffering from GI tract problems assume that increased fiber will help the situation, but this is not always true. If diarrhea is your primary IBS symptom, increasing fiber intake may actually worsen the problem. The primary culprits among high-fiber foods are beans and an overload of fruits and vegetables. Instead, try a small increase in whole-grain wheat bread or crackers, or even a bulking agent such as Metamucil, to help improve diarrhea symptoms safely without the overwhelming effects some natural high-fiber foods can have. If gas and bloating are your problems, avoid certain fibrous foods as much as possible. However, if constipation is a regular symptom, increasing the amount of fiber in your diet would certainly help. Foods high in fiber include wheat, bran, and oats, as well as vegetables and fruits. Gas-producing fibrous foods include beans and cruciferous vegetables, such as brussels sprouts, cauliflower, and cabbage. (Caffeine-heavy drinks, such as coffee and sodas, are also likely to produce gas.)

Spices

Some people can't get enough spice, and others don't like either the flavor or the physical reaction they get from spices. Many IBS sufferers have trouble with spices, and these flavoring agents may also aggravate dyspepsia. Consume the following spices cautiously, in small amounts, to determine whether they have negative effects on you:

- Black pepper
- Chili powder
- Chili peppers
- Cloves
- Curry powder
- Garlic
- Ginger
- Hot sauce
- Mustard seed
- Nutmeg
- Spicy barbecue sauce

Caffeine

Caffeine can wreak havoc with the IBS sufferer. Found in coffee, tea, soft drinks, and chocolate, as well as over-the-counter diet aids and pain relievers, caffeine works against the IBS patient in three primary ways:

1. It stimulates the GI tract, triggering diarrhea and cramping and promoting symptoms of heartburn and dyspepsia.

2. It stimulates brain and heart activity, creating symptoms of anxiety and panic, which can actually create those emotions in you (see the discussion in chapter two).
3. It disturbs sleep, and the loss of sleep contributes to stress and anxiety.

If you feel you must have caffeine, limit it to one cup of coffee or tea a day, and do not consume it on an empty stomach. However, at least while you're getting your health under control, the best idea is to eliminate it altogether. Do so over a period of days, because stopping caffeine all of a sudden—particularly if you consume a good deal daily—can lead to withdrawal-induced headaches.

Pinpointing Your Troublesome Foods

Once you have initially determined which foods may be involved in your bouts of IBS, begin the process of removing them from your diet little by little, to see if some improvement results. Now is also the time to eliminate some bad eating habits that likely contribute to your problem.

A good way to begin is by eliminating those foods that have the least nutritional value and that seem to instigate the most disruptive attacks. Do as much as you can comfortably do. Not only does eliminating a great number foods at one time pose a real hardship, but it may also present a less accurate picture of just which foods are causing your problems.

Good foods to eliminate include

- Fast food
- Foods that contain both high fat and high dairy content, such as ice cream and cheddar cheese

➤ Raw vegetables
➤ Beans and other gas-producing foods

While you eliminate a potential troublemaking food, note whether a particular eating habit causes you distress. Perhaps you always have a cup of coffee before eating anything in the morning, or you have a habit of eating your lunch while returning phone calls. How you eat can be as important as what you eat when gastrointestinal problems are involved.

Eating quickly involves gulping vast quantities of air, which can lead to gas—both belching and flatulence—and stomach distension. Moreover, the intestinal tract is a complex and highly sensitive organ (see the discussion in chapter one). Abuse or overload it, and you will undoubtedly pay a price.

Change one troublesome eating habit at a time. For instance, rather than eating lunch at your desk, take it outside, or to a quiet, empty space somewhere in your office building. Even if you allow yourself only twenty uninterrupted minutes to sit quietly, eat, and begin to digest in a peaceful atmosphere, you may find it makes a big difference. If you think you can't spare those minutes away from the phones or paperwork, ask yourself how much time you may have to spend in the rest room if you don't, or how much longer a task may take if you're distracted by a pain in your gut.

Another habit to avoid is skipping meals altogether. A too-empty stomach, like a too-full one, puts a real strain on the digestive tract. Consistent and thoughtful eating habits are key to improving IBS symptoms.

What to Eat Instead

Eliminating foods is one thing, but you might be asking, "What do I eat instead?" Despite the fact that we live in the richest nation in the world, and through miracles of agriculture, shipping, catalog shopping, and Internet shopping we can (for a price) buy any food we wish at any time, many of us are in food ruts. For those who don't cook, or who cook very little, the idea of changing from a diet based on fast food and takeout seems almost impossible. But take heart—you can make changes to eliminate trigger foods without turning your life upside down. In the next sections, I offer some food swaps—whether you're starting from fast food or a typical home-cooked diet— that can set you on the road to feeling better.

Fast-Food Substitutions

Except for the food purists among us, everyone enjoys the occasional burger on the run. Unfortunately, for some it has become a way of life. However, even they can improve their diet with these alternative choices at the fast-food counter.

Breakfast

If you start your day at a fast-food restaurant, here are some choices to try.

- Instead of breakfast sandwiches, opt for pancakes, and specify no butter. Have a side of poached or scrambled eggs to add protein, and skip the bacon. If toast is available, have it with jelly instead of butter, and choose wheat bread if you suffer from constipation or gas. White bread might set better if you have severe diarrhea.

- If you have the breakfast sandwich, choose thin-sliced ham, rather than sausage and bacon, which are generally fattier. Try ordering the vegetarian sandwich with only egg and cheese, or simply a poached egg and bread. Breakfast sandwiches made on an English muffin are infinitely preferable to those made on a croissant because of the fat difference.
- French fries or hash browns are best left behind the counter.
- Skip the coffee, and have a cup of weak tea. Herb tea is generally the best choice. Make it a habit to carry one or two bags of your favorite blend with you whenever possible because herb tea is not always available in restaurants.

Lunch and Dinner

- At fast-food restaurants, grilled chicken is the best possible choice.
- If you suffer from constipation, try eating the chicken sandwich without the bread, and add a side salad with oil-and-vinegar dressing.
- If diarrhea is a common problem, forgo the salad, and add a cup of soup (not cream-based) to your meal.
- If you must have a burger, the most acceptable choice is a hamburger without additional fat in

the form of cheese, mayonnaise-based sauce, or the like (ketchup or mustard is fine).

➤ At burger restaurants, avoid fried fish at all costs. Although popular wisdom holds that fish is a healthy choice, in fast-food restaurants the fried-fish sandwich is often the highest-fat item on the menu.

Delicatessen Substitutions

Although the deli is certainly an easier place to assemble a healthy meal than a fast-food stand, you still must use diligence to avoid some common triggers of IBS.

Breakfast
Many people think a bagel or muffin is a healthy choice, but the truth is that they can be laden with fat. Instead, try the following:

➤ Ask for wheat toast with a side of jam.
➤ See whether a low-fat bran muffin is available.
➤ If you want a bagel, try it with a tiny amount of cream cheese, and add tomato and lox, also in small amounts.
➤ Get a small side of fruit salad.
➤ Consider starting your day with a turkey sandwich—it's not conventional, but it's healthy and easily digested. Order it without a mayonnaise dressing (mustard is fine) and without cheese. If diarrhea is a problem, reduce or eliminate lettuce, tomatoes, onions, sprouts, and the like from the sandwich.

Lunch

→ A sliced turkey or chicken sandwich (without mayonnaise or cheese) on wheat, rye, or pumpernickel, with whatever vegetables and toppings you can comfortably enjoy, is the best option. Try it on wheat bread with mustard.

→ Avoid mayonnaise-laden side salads, such as potato and macaroni. Have a fruit or green salad instead.

→ If you're dying for a tuna sandwich, ask for no extra mayonnaise on the bread.

→ Avoid fatty sandwich specials, such as meatballs, hoagies, or grilled sandwiches.

→ A cup of soup may be a good addition to lunch, although bean soups may cause problems for some sufferers and cream-based soups should definitely be avoided.

→ Skip the potato chips and French fries.

Pizza Parlor Substitutions

→ If pizza is your choice, ask for thin crust rather than thick.

→ Choose a plain or vegetable pizza rather than meat.

→ Ask for no cheese or a reduced amount of cheese on your pizza.

→ If diarrhea isn't an issue for you, order a large salad, with dressing on the side so that you can add an amount that both your taste buds can enjoy and your digestive tract can accept. Then eat only a small slice of pizza.

Chicken and Other Entrée Takeout Substitutions

If takeout involves full meals, here are some general adjustments that may help.

- Choose roasted or grilled, rather than fried, lean cuts of chicken, beef, lamb, pork, fish, or shellfish.
- Ask whether vegetables are available steamed without butter or oil, and if so choose that method.
- Choose a baked potato dry, with sour cream or butter on the side, so that you may add a small amount to enjoy without instigating symptoms. Try nonfat yogurt, salsa, or chutney as an alternative to or in combination with fatty toppings to reduce your fat intake.
- Avoid gravy.

Chinese Food Substitutions

Chinese food offers a number of possibilities for an IBS-friendly order.

- Ask the restaurant to prepare dishes with a minimum of oil.
- Substitute white-meat chicken for fattier dark meat.
- Always opt for steamed white or brown rice rather than fried rice.
- Avoid fatty choices such as spring rolls or fried wonton.

✦ Skip spicy Szechuan dishes in favor of milder Mandarin or Cantonese entrées.

Mexican Food Substitutions

✦ An order of fajitas, a chicken enchilada without guacamole or sour cream, or a soft chicken taco is least likely to cause problems.
✦ Ask the cook to hold the sour cream and guacamole.
✦ Opt for mild salsa, and have it on the side.
✦ Although it's not easy, forgo the taco chips and hard taco shells. Ask for a side of steamed corn tortillas instead.

Home-Cooked Meal Substitutions

Cooking at home offers you endless opportunities to prepare dishes you like in a way that won't exacerbate your symptoms. Here are a few options to consider.

Breakfast

✦ When possible, opt for low-fat, high-fiber foods such as oatmeal or bran cereal with skim milk. Avoid whole milk.
✦ If you must have eggs, soft-boil or poach them. Avoid choices that involve cooking in fat.
✦ Skip the traditional bacon or sausage. If you miss them, try the low-fat turkey versions.
✦ Pancakes and waffles can be a good part of a low-fat breakfast. Skip the butter, add some fruit, and drizzle on a small amount of syrup. Try a poached egg on the side to add protein.

→ If you must have coffee, drink decaffeinated. Tea is a better choice, however, because even decaf is irritating to some IBS sufferers.

Lunch

The more often you can prepare a healthy lunch for yourself, the better.

→ Sandwiches (without cheese, mayo, or other fatty dressings) and low-fat soups are always good options. Try to keep easily tolerated low-fat cold cuts such as chicken or turkey in the house.

→ When you prepare an IBS-friendly dinner, make an extra amount, if possible, and have the leftovers for lunch.

Dinner

→ When constipation is an issue, try to include a salad that is rich in a variety of greens along with raw vegetables, such as carrots, celery, and mushrooms, and cooked vegetables, such as spinach and green beans, that aren't likely to promote gas.

→ Homemade soups are an excellent source of quick and nonirritating food. Cook up a big batch of turkey vegetable soup on a Sunday, and freeze it in small batches to eat later.

→ Eat fish and chicken rather than red meat as much as possible. When eating meat, go for lean cuts. Pork and lamb are preferable to beef. Trim the fat before cooking.

→ Cook dishes such as stew in advance and chill

them in the refrigerator so that you can easily remove the hardened fat on the top. The remaining lean meat and cooked vegetables are far less likely to trigger IBS. Make enough to reheat for an easy, healthy lunch.

➤ Make steamed rice or a dry or lightly dressed baked potato as a side dish.

➤ If you prefer mashed potatoes, make them with low-fat or nonfat milk and a little fat-free chicken stock for flavor.

➤ Avoid Tabasco sauce, spicy salsa, curry powder, and excessive salt and pepper, as they can upset digestion.

The Right Environment for Eating

It's not just what but how you eat that matters. Here are some simple tips for making mealtimes pleasant and positive.

➤ Don't eat on the run. Gulping food while standing up, running out, or driving the car wreaks havoc on the digestive tract. Get up fifteen minutes earlier to have a quiet breakfast. Wait until the kids are napping to sit and have some lunch.

➤ Sit down for dinner. Somewhere in the last decade the notion of dinnertime was sacrificed in many families to soccer schedules, late nights at the office, and microwave dinners in front of the TV. Dinner should be a relaxing time. If you're part of a family, bring everyone together for at least a half hour of shared food and conversation as many times a week as possible.

→ If you can't gather your family for a calm, sit-down meal, try not to eat while the others are grabbing a chaotic meal. Instead, have a cup of tea and talk to your kids and spouse; eat your own dinner quietly by yourself before or after they do.

→ If you're living on your own, make yourself an appetizing and attractive plate of food, sit down in a quiet, comfortable, pleasant place, and slowly enjoy your dinner.

→ Don't eat large meals late at night—your body's attempt to digest them can disrupt your sleep patterns.

→ Don't use straws to drink—they increase the amount of air you ingest and may cause gas.

→ Avoid sucking hard candy and chewing gum—both can lead you to swallow air and suffer discomfort from gas.

These are just a few ideas for simple ways to modify your daily diet and eating patterns. The more aware you become of your food and behavior triggers, the easier it will be for you to modify your meals and habits to avoid them.

Diet for Children with IBS

For the child who has been diagnosed with IBS, the predominant symptom is usually either diarrhea or pain. When pain is predominant, the IBS is characterized by cramping that is subsequently relieved by passing stools or gas. The primary treatment, whichever symptom is prevalent, is a dietary change to increased fiber and reduced fat. Use of even over-the-counter medications such as laxatives should be kept to a minimum with children. Older children may be able to learn some stress-reduction techniques (see chapter six), but the best way to address the symptoms is by helping the child to eat an IBS-friendly diet and thus gain control over the diarrhea, gas, and pain.

Food Allergies

Some people are allergic to certain foods, although many supposed allergies are intolerances (see chapter four). In reviewing your diary, if you find that one or two foods bring about a particularly immediate and violent reaction, you may want to be tested by your doctor for a food allergy. If you are found to be allergic, you will likely need to eliminate that food from your diet as completely as possible. If you are not allergic but rather intolerant of that food, you can enjoy it occasionally without concern about an intense reaction.

Two tests are used to determine food allergies. The most common is the scratch test, in which a small amount of the allergen is placed on your skin, and then a needle prick or scratch is made at that spot to allow a minute amount to penetrate the skin. If an allergy in fact exists, the scratched area will soon react with redness or swelling or both. Scratch tests are not entirely accurate, and two over-the-counter medications can inhibit their accuracy—

antihistamines and topical creams containing steroids. To ensure that your test is as accurate as possible, avoid both these medications for several days before seeing the doctor.

The other test to determine food allergies is the radioallergosorbent test (RAST), a blood test. It is more expensive and generally no more accurate than the skin test, but it may be preferable for patients who have the following concerns:

- They will suffer an extreme and unpleasant allergic reaction to the skin test
- The skin test will be painful because they have a condition or disease that makes their skin extremely sensitive
- They have dermatographism, a condition in which hives result if the skin is touched or scratched
- They will suffer adverse effects if they stop taking antihistamines

If allergies are not found by testing, you may have a food intolerance, a milder condition. To pinpoint the culprit, begin reintroducing one by one the foods you had eliminated from your diet.

Combating Fear of Food

For most people, changes in diet offer at least some relief. It's important, however, not to begin to view food as a negative. There's no reason you can't continue to enjoy food and all the social pleasures that can accompany it. Unfortunately, some people who suffer from IBS stop getting any pleasure from mealtime and, in the worst-case scenario, literally develop a fear of food.

When eating makes a person sick, she may respond by skipping meals or eating only at home or in private. She may avoid social situations that involve food, or stay only briefly before or after a meal to prevent the embarrassment of having to run to the toilet or excuse herself because of gastrointestinal pain. Over time, just the thought of eating can cause her stomach to seize up and cramp in nervous anticipation of what a meal may bring. Some people who suffer from this fear become virtual hermits, prisoners of their gastric troubles.

The diabolical nature of this cycle is that the stress brought on by the thought of eating is likely to trigger IBS symptoms as much as or more than the food itself. For people in this condition, reintroducing foods, discussed next, is especially important. Once you've determined some of the food triggers of IBS, you need to discover which foods you can reintroduce into your diet and in what quantities.

Reintroducing Foods in Your Diet

When you've identified foods that trigger your symptoms, eliminate those foods from your diet for two to six weeks. There are two reasons for this: First, it gives you time to determine whether other factors linked to that food may have been involved in the trigger. For instance, suppose that you always had eggs and toast in the morning while you were getting the kids off to school. Is it the eggs or the hassle with the kids that has your digestive tract in knots? Second, some foods may affect you only cumulatively. You need to remove them completely from your diet so that you can reintroduce them to determine whether you can eat them occasionally. Altering your diet over a period of time gives you a better chance to evaluate your symptoms and determine whether food, stress, or a combination has been causing your problems.

If you have become food phobic, the food reintroduction process is particularly important, and you need to use stress-reduction techniques along with your meals (see chapter six). You are, in some ways, reintroducing all foods into your diet. If you have had an extremely severe IBS attack (or any other severe gastric disturbance), you might first want to try what specialists call the *BRAT diet:* bananas, rice, applesauce, and toast. Once you've been able to digest that, and your symptoms have subsided, begin slowly reintroducing other foods, slowly eating small portions throughout the day in a calm, quiet environment.

Begin with the plainest foods possible. The following can be tolerated by almost everyone.

- A small amount of natural fruit spread added to your toast
- Scrambled eggs cooked with nonfat spray
- Canned fruit
- Baked potato
- Steamed rice
- Roasted or steamed white-meat turkey or chicken
- Nonfat yogurt

- Low-fat whole-wheat crackers
- Ripe bananas, pears, kiwis, peaches, and nectarines
- Cooked green beans, peas, mushrooms, spinach, zucchini, and carrots
- Nonfat vegetable and chicken broth

Once you can eat these comfortably, begin expanding your diet. Reintroduce foods one item at a time, eating small amounts in a relaxed setting. Remember that some foods trigger a reaction only if consumed too often; they cause no problem on the first day you eat them but do trigger symptoms when you continue to eat them for three or four consecutive days.

While you keep track of the foods that trigger your IBS symptoms, note which foods you can almost always eat comfortably. When you're going through periods of stress and upset, fall back on those foods to help keep your symptoms to a minimum. If you have a favorite soup or entrée that always tastes good and leaves you feeling good, make a big batch and freeze it in meal-size quantities so that you'll have a quick, easy meal when you need it most.

Obviously, although food may be an IBS trigger for you, you cannot eliminate it from your life. But you'll find that you don't need to do that to be able to live more comfortably with IBS.

CHAPTER SIX

Stress Strategies

S tress is the primary trigger of IBS symptoms. Limit-
ing or avoiding stressful situations, whenever possible, and finding new and better ways of coping with
the stress you cannot eliminate are the best prescriptions
for living better with IBS.

The first step is to understand what, and who, may be
causing you stress. As Dr. Hans Selye identified, stress is
extremely subjective—a situation that helps one person to
thrive, or spurs him on to succeed, can be disastrous for
another. That's why it's important to start a journal chron-
icling the events of your day and your gastrointestinal reactions to them. Clearly, this diary requires a more
complex and thoughtful recording process than the food
diary described in chapter five, and it may seem odd at
first to take time out when you already feel stressed and
overwhelmed to add one more task—making a record of
what's happening. Actually, the effort will lead not only
to the long-term benefit of better understanding your
stress but also to a significant short-term benefit: taking a
moment to really focus on what's upsetting you and to

record the event can help you take a breath and get perspective. Stress and upset can, as we all know, quickly snowball if not addressed. Obviously, if stress is occurring in the middle of a soccer game you're coaching, or a conference with your boss, you'll need to wait to record what happened and your reaction to it. Try to take mental notes, along with a deep breath to remind yourself that this moment will pass!

Keeping a Stress Diary

To track your day accurately, you need to consider not just the events that trigger stress but also how you were feeling before they happened. Keep track of the following:

- How did you sleep? Were you able to fall asleep quickly last night, or did it take you a long time? Did you find yourself playing over the events of the previous day?
- How did you feel about the day when you woke up? Were you already stressed? Looking forward to the day? Feeling focused? Feeling overwhelmed?
- How were you feeling physically upon waking up? Was your GI tract relaxed and functioning normally or was it already in knots?
- What was the first stress of the day? What was your physical response? How did you feel after the event? Record the answers for each stress of the day.

- Did you recover reasonably quickly after a stressful event, or did the stresses of the day seem to pile up? Did your feeling of being stressed escalate throughout the day?
- What was your digestive system's physical response after each stressful event? How long did it last? How intense was it?
- How did you feel at the end of the day?

In addition to events, you need to consider honestly how people affect you. It may be difficult, but consider how the following people make you feel:

- Your spouse
- Your children
- Your boss
- Your co-workers
- Your neighbors
- Your friends

The idea in recording your feelings is not to assign blame or suggest that people need to be eliminated from your life for you to feel well again, but rather to understand how the ways in which you interact with others may be affecting you. It's also important to consider how your expectations of yourself might make your dealings with others difficult. For instance, are you someone who feels that your way is the best way? If this is the case, you might find that a number of stresses in your dealings with people involve your own inability to let go.

Ranking and Dealing with Stressors

Once you have taken a detailed look at the stresses that trigger your IBS problems, begin evaluating and ranking them, starting with those that you can eliminate or control simply, continuing with those that you'll need to make some effort to deal with or change, and ending with those that are beyond your control—a fact that you must accept if you are to make peace and live comfortably with them.

The next sections discuss these three ranks of stressors, offering examples and solutions to help you deal with and alleviate them as common triggers of IBS.

Easily Reduced Stressors

Some stressors that you identify you can greatly diminish or eliminate entirely with a bit of attention and planning. I'm not suggesting that these stressors do not wreak havoc with your life. There are certainly times and circumstances in which they feel completely unmanageable. But, unlike some stressors, these can usually be greatly diminished, or even eliminated from daily life if you give them some attention and planning.

Life's Little Irritants
Certain little things go wrong day after day. They may seem minor, but they regularly cost you time and peace of mind. Often they are things you promise yourself you'll

address—only to put them on the back burner until they cause problems again. Consider these common irritants and a few ways to address and diminish them. I understand that some of the solutions may seem exceedingly obvious to you. I'm not suggesting that you haven't thought of them already. Rather, this list is meant to be a prompt for you to do the little things you've been putting off. The very fact that these solutions are simplistic will, I hope, lead you to the conclusion that there's no excuse for not doing them.

Where did I leave my keys? It seems like a little thing, but think about how frustrating it is—the annoyance of looking for them, the anger at yourself for losing them again, the stress of running late because of the time spent searching for them. Each of these is a classic IBS trigger.

Solve this problem with a two-pronged approach: First, pound a nail into the wall near the door where you first come into the house (yes, a fancy hook would be nice, but how long would it be before you remembered to buy one?), and get yourself into the habit of hanging them there the minute you walk through the door. Second, make several extra sets for both house and car. Leave one at the office, another in a safe place in the house. This way, you always know where at least one set is, and you can be on your way, one stressor lighter.

There's the phone again. So many of us now have a variety of ways for people to reach us—home phone, cell phone, beeper, e-mail, and fax. But what was supposed to be a convenience has, in many ways, become an intrusion that is more than a little out of hand. It is hard to stay focused, and calmly and easily complete tasks when confronted by constant ringing and beeping. Unless the bulk of your calls are work related, a lot of communications probably don't need your attention that minute and merely cause unnecessary and upsetting disruptions in your schedule. Instead of responding immediately to every call, use your voice mail and answering machine to best advantage. Let them pick up your messages, and then use your discretion about what's urgent and what's not. Allot yourself a certain time each day to return friends' calls or make appointments.

Perhaps most important, *make mealtimes phone-free.* Unless you have some urgent reason not to disable the phone, such as a sick relative or a dependent child who needs to be able to reach you at any moment, turn the ringer off for at least fifteen minutes (more if you can), and eat your meals in peace. At first this may seem hard, and you may be nervous about missing a call, but it won't take long for you to enjoy having control over the phone rather than vice versa. As a bonus, think of all the telemarketers you'll miss! If the idea of turning off the phone seems unthinkable, ask yourself this question: Did you have a pager or cell phone five years ago? Until recently we all lived just fine without instant communication, and we were probably happier and healthier for it.

What happened to that bill (or other important paper)? While some people are well organized, most of us bring the mail in, drop it somewhere, and plan to deal with it later. During a hurried cleanup, we stuff bills and papers into a drawer or put them on another pile. Later, when it's time to find them, a lengthy and irritating search ensues. Worse, out of sight really may mean out of mind until an upsetting late fee or phone call reminds us of a forgotten bill. No person suffering a stress disorder needs to endure this irritant.

Find one place to accumulate bills and papers, even if it's just a shoebox. Too often we wait for a perfect solution to a simple problem. You don't need a designer mail holder or ornate basket to get your life in order. You simply need to get in the habit of putting things in one place. That way, even if you can't look through them immediately, you'll know where to look when you need them.

Also take a minute to write on a daily calendar a reminder to mail each of your bills seven days before its due date. That way, you won't rely on the visual cue of seeing a bill. Instead, you'll begin a routine of paying on time that will become second nature and eliminate some ongoing stress.

Clearly, other similar daily issues can be tackled without much effort. Do one every other day, and then take a minute to applaud your own efforts. Taking the time to acknowledge what you've accomplished, as opposed to scolding yourself for what has yet to be done, is also a great way to decrease your stress.

Household Chores and the Disease to Please

While everyone has chores, this section is particularly dedicated to the woman who feels she must do it all, and do it perfectly. This is the kind of person who, as we discussed in chapter three, believes that she will somehow be less liked, and even less of a person, if she asks for help, says no, or asks others for things. When it comes to chores, this woman is probably overwhelmed by laundry, grocery shopping, errands, and cleaning while not doing the one thing that could make her life much easier: delegating.

Delegating

Delegate—that is the message of this section. Look at the section of your diary of daily stressors that involves household chores, and ask yourself the following questions:

- ➤ Which of these chores could be assigned to someone else in the house?
- ➤ Which of these chores could be done less often?
- ➤ Concerning the chores that could be delegated, why haven't you done so before? Do you feel guilty about asking your mate or your children to do something they don't enjoy? Are you afraid they'll be angry or not like you anymore? Or is it another common reason—that you don't feel the job will be done "right" if somebody else does it?

When considering the notion of doing it right, I am reminded of a woman I saw on a daytime talk show. She vacuumed the carpet at least once a day and took extreme care to put track marks into it to show that it had just been cleaned. Of course the minute her husband or children stepped on the rug, her handiwork was ruined, and she had to do it all over again. Somehow, her notion of who she was and the job she did running the house was tied up in that carpet. Imagine the stress she felt watching the carpet, waiting for the first footprint to ruin it. Imagine the upset she felt at whoever made that step and her nervous need to grab the vacuum and make things right again.

While this woman was an extreme case, most women—if honest—can see something of themselves in her. Tied up in our notions of being a good wife, or mother, or woman is the perfectly kept house—visible proof to the world, not to mention the neighbors, that we are doing the right thing, taking good care of the family, keeping on top of things. Of course, the dark side to all this is that, rather than taking care of the family, we may actually be creating unnecessary discord. Imagine the fights that must have occurred about that carpet. After all, how can family members feel happy in a home where they can't walk freely? And, by constantly focusing on how we look to the world, we put ourselves in a position of constantly being judged—even if the judgment is in our minds. That creates a great deal of stress.

So go through your household chores, and think of how to best delegate them. If you have children, think of what they can do. Children like to participate—a five-year-old can feed the dog, sort socks, or take out a light amount of garbage. Lower your expectations a bit. The tub should be clean, but you don't need to see your reflection in it!

If you have roommates, have each of them and yourself make a list of household chores. Then sit down together to divide the tasks fairly. Make a schedule and stick to it. If you live on your own and find yourself compulsively cleaning, ask yourself why. Are you expecting your perfect mate to walk in unexpectedly and fall in love with your sparkling faucets? Are you still being ruled by the voice of your mother, even though you no longer live with her? Set a schedule and time limits for your housework, and stick to it. Make a conscious effort to make your home a place to relax in and enjoy.

Whether you live alone or with others, if you can afford it, consider hiring a housekeeper who comes in once a week to take care of the basics. This relatively small cost might leave you free for other things and reduce your stress. If you've been seeing the doctor, missing work, and in other ways losing income, having a housekeeper might be not only a healthy choice but also an economically advantageous one.

Another chore that may eat up a lot of your time is grocery shopping. Keep track of the things you most often run out of, and try to stock up to minimize shopping trips. If you're the parent of teenagers who can drive (or there's a market safely within bicycling distance) don't hesitate to send them on last-minute grocery runs. If, like me, you actually enjoy going to the market, do it late in the evening when the store is quiet, the lines are short, and you can take your time, thinking, daydreaming, being extra careful to choose foods that both taste good to you and are easy on your digestion.

Once you start to delegate and free up some time, the trick is to use it productively and constructively. One of the very best things you can do to decrease the effects of stress and improve your overall health is to exercise.

Stress and Exercise

When I talk about exercise, I'm not picturing a room full of perfectly clad body worshippers spinning or stair-stepping or doing aerobics to loud music and the rapidly barked instructions of a flawless instructor (although, if that relaxes you, go for it!). Exercise should be something that calms and centers you, something that can be done with a minimum of preparation, and something that helps both your body and your mind. If you enjoy structured exercise and learning a new skill, yoga, tai chi, or a formal exercise program is an excellent choice, offering benefits for both physical and mental health. If you would rather get exercise in less structured ways, gardening, playing with children, and walking offer possibilities.

Yoga

Yoga is an ancient series of exercises that strengthens muscles, improves posture, and increases flexibility and range of motion. It has been proven to increase heart efficiency, lower blood pressure, promote relaxation, reduce stress, and allay anxiety. It also improves sleep, concentration, and—of particular importance to the IBS patient—digestion.

Physicians have recommended yoga for everything from cancer to arthritis to migraines. Yoga does not, by itself, offer a cure for any disease, but it is a contributing factor in Dr. Dean Ornish's well-known and successful program of diet and exercise to reverse heart disease.

If you would like to take yoga, classes are generally available at private studios, gyms, recreation centers, and community colleges. Sessions include breathing exercises, body postures, and meditation. Many yoga studios offer other advice about living a healthy life, including nutritional recommendations. Classes vary in degree from gentle introductory postures to the strenuous, intensely aerobic instruction favored by many in the Hollywood community. The benefits of yoga can be enhanced by meditation. For traditional practitioners, yoga is as much a spiritual pursuit as a physical one.

To find the yoga class that is right for you, observe or participate in several different ones. You can also rent yoga videos, although, if you're not physically fit or if you have any back or other joint problem, attempting the postures without supervision is not recommended.

Tai Chi Chuan

Like other ancient Chinese practices, tai chi chuan (or tai chi) is intended to harmonize the body's *yin* and *yang* and release its vital energy flow. Tai chi was derived from the martial arts and must be taught by an experienced instructor whose background is in those arts.

In clinical trials, tai chi has been proven to reduce blood pressure and heart rate. It improves strength and muscle tone, enhances range of motion and flexibility, improves balance and coordination, and, because it is a weight-bearing exercise, improves bone density and diminishes risk of osteoporosis. A gentle, low-impact exercise, it offers particular benefits to older people and those who are out of shape, since it promotes wellness without risk of injury. Even the disabled can employ and reap the advantages of tai chi—in fact, movements have been adapted successfully for people in wheelchairs.

Because tai chi promotes the ability to concentrate and focus on breathing and movement to the exclusion of all else, it can greatly help IBS sufferers to manage stress and stress-induced symptoms, while it contributes to their general well-being.

Many community centers and colleges offer tai chi instruction. You might also inquire about instruction at martial arts studios. Observe a class before making a long-term commitment—the instructor should communicate clearly and patiently so that learning tai chi is an enjoyable and beneficial experience.

Exercise Classes and Workouts

Most communities offer exercise classes at the local gym, YMCA, or community college. If you prefer to work out alone, videotaped exercise instruction is available. Working out with weights—focusing on precision and slowly building strength—can also be calming and rewarding. It's important to do these exercises correctly; a single session with a personal trainer, supplemented by instructional videos, can help you both prevent injuries and maximize the benefits you'll obtain from exercise.

Gardening

You can get excellent exercise for both mind and body by gardening. It offers a good physical workout and the mental and spiritual benefits that come from working with the earth. Remember that gardening can be surprisingly hard on the body if you don't use the proper form and tools. Gloves, knee pads, a workbench, a hat to protect you from the sun—all are important to keep gardening comfortable and enjoyable.

Playing with Children

Another great exercise for both body and mind is playing with kids, your own or somebody else's, whether you join in a game of tag or do something active, one on one. Laughing and playing with children is a wonderful way to get out of your own head and have fun, with all the resultant mental benefits added to the physical exertion required to keep up with the kids.

Walking

No other exercise is better for you than the one you can do anytime, anywhere, if you're blessed enough to have the use of your legs: walking. Walking may be the most natural form of exercise imaginable, but you wouldn't know it from the articles, videos, and instructors detailing how to do it. Chin up, arms bent and pumping, heel-toe-heel-toe—no doubt, these instructions provide optimum cardiac benefit, but they may also take some of the fun out of your daily stroll and diminish some of its less obvious stress relievers.

I love to walk in my Hollywood Hills neighborhood. Clearly the uphill climb does good things for my lower body, but it's the benefit to my mood that I really miss when I can't take my usual outing. No matter how tense I am, by the time I've enjoyed the many distractions of my walk—observing the improvements on my neighbors' property; greeting the local dogs; or hearing snatches of music and conversation floating out of open windows—I've relaxed and begun to find some perspective on my troubles and my day.

This is the kind of walk I'm suggesting—the kind that frees your mind as well as moves your body. The walk can last fifteen minutes or an hour. It can take place indoors or out. All it requires is good shoes; comfortable clothes that are appropriate for the weather; some water, and, if your walk is going to be long, a snack.

To really reap the calming benefits of a good walk, include the following:

- Seek solitude. This is not the time for rehashing problems, comparing symptoms, dishing the dirt, or trying to adjust to someone else's mood. Make your walk a time to let your mind wander, and allow yourself to be happily distracted. If you are just not comfortable being alone, try to find someone of like mind—someone willing to be quiet and open to the sights and sounds around the two of you.
- Put the concept of exercise out of your mind. Forget about heart rate, weight loss, and all the other buzzwords that have become associated with aerobic activity. Instead, focus on the pleasure and good fortune you enjoy from being able to put one foot in front of the other. Dawdle when you feel like it, and move faster when you feel a burst of energy. Take a moment to appreciate the engineering genius that is the human body, as well as the gift of your ability to take a good walk.
- Look for beauty. Even the grittiest urban neighborhood has undiscovered treasures that most people pass by every day. When you start

noticing the unexpected rose bush, the beautiful antique ironwork on an otherwise rundown building, the loveliness of kids playing in a schoolyard, you stop focusing on—and fretting over—your life's everyday problems and as a result feel more relaxed and less stressed.

➤ Visit someplace you've been meaning to go. It could be the beach, or a block of historic buildings, or a park you haven't been to since childhood. Walk, take your time, and really look around. Not only will you have a wonderful and relaxing outing, but you'll also fulfill a wish—maybe a small one, but rewarding nonetheless. You will have one more positive experience that helps reduce stress and promotes well-being.

➤ Walk like a child. Kids see things we don't. Partly it's their size—the hedge we tower over offers children hiding places, potential pets, and a wealth of stimuli for active imaginations. But more than that, they don't have our pressures of time or responsibility. If you don't remember how children view the world, take one on a walk with you. Don't pull her along; adjust to her pace. She'll teach you a great deal about the joys of staying in the moment.

➤ Leave the Walkman at home. Your walk isn't just about exercising your body, it's also about the relaxation that comes from keeping your mind and eyes open, enjoying the peacefulness of a neighborhood in the early morning or the hustle and bustle of the afternoon. Headphones, even those playing your favorite music or books on tape, keep the world out. You then lose the many delights and distractions it has to offer.

Whenever possible, start your day with a walk. You'll be amazed at the benefits you reap all day from a peaceful fifteen-minute morning stroll.

Stress and Psychotherapy

When stress overwhelms you despite your best efforts on your own, therapy may be called for. Having a trained and objective listener can help you to put your life and problems into perspective, and perspective—or lack of it—is often a primary cause of stress and anxiety.

Studies have shown that therapy offers tremendous benefits for the IBS sufferer. A joint study by the University of North Carolina and the University of Toronto, reported in *Chatelaine* (January 1999), confirms that the hypersensitive gut of the IBS sufferer reacts more strongly to stressors than the digestive tract of the average person. All of us have a mind/gut response to some degree, but for IBS patients the symptoms of cramping, diarrhea, and the like are more frequent and severe. Research has found that many IBS sufferers are unable to identify what causes them stress. Once stressors are identified, patients learn to improve their reactions to stress by avoiding a tendency to jump to conclusions, engage in perfectionism, or view problems as overwhelming or catastrophic. In short, therapy helps them gain perspective; perspective goes a long way toward relieving stress; and reduction of stress relieves the symptoms of IBS.

Guilt plays a role in the stress felt by some women with IBS. Psychologist Brenda Toner of the Centre for Research in Women's Health (connected to the Women's College Hospital and the University of Toronto) says traditional gender roles contribute to the problems of women with IBS, particularly working women. "Society gives women mixed messages. Be focused and competitive, but take care of others without complaint. That's unhealthy."

Even if you identify stressors by analyzing your daily journal, you may not begin to feel real improvement. Many people need professional help in overcoming the guilt they feel for simply looking after themselves instead of putting everyone else first. Going through the motions of taking a few minutes for yourself won't reduce your IBS symptoms if those moments are really spent beating yourself up for not doing something else. A therapist can help you understand that you don't just need but also deserve to have your own time, your own needs, and your own desires. Once you really believe you're entitled to these things, the stress of self-imposed pressures and perfectionism is enormously diminished.

With perspective and an improved sense of self-worth, you will begin to take control over your life and health. In a May 15, 2000, interview for Radio National's "Health Report," Professor Douglas Drossman of the University of North Carolina at Chapel Hill, an IBS specialist, summed up the benefits of treatments that help people manage their pain better. "If [people] perceive that [they] can control . . . and can decrease [their] symptoms, even if [they] actually can't, if [they] feel [they] can, those individuals did better one year later than those who felt they had no control over their symptoms."

The sense of control you can gain from having the tools for handling stress can have unexpected, practical benefits. For instance, when one member of Dr. Toner's study began participating in the research, she hadn't gone to the movies in fifteen years because she felt so self-conscious about her many trips to the restroom. Four months into therapy, she attended a film festival and saw sixteen movies in ten days!

If you think therapy may be good for you, you can track down an appropriate professional in several places. First, speak to your general practitioner or gastroenterologist. She may know of a therapeutic professional with special interest or training in the area of IBS or the relationship between stress and physical illness.

If you don't have a regular practitioner, contact the gastroenterology department of your local hospital. Personnel there may be able to offer referrals, or on occasion even be aware of studies (such as the ones cited in this section) that are seeking participants.

If this avenue isn't helpful, check in the yellow pages under "Mental Health Services" for county referrals and assistance. County assistance can be especially helpful for those on a limited income. Under "Psychologists" you'll find both referral services and individual counselors listing their specialties. Rather than picking a name at random from the book, go through a referral service, or visit an established clinic with a variety of practitioners. Don't be embarrassed or ashamed to talk to family and friends; they

may be able to offer a referral or the name of a health professional who can offer one. You may learn that someone
else in your family has been suffering from a similar problem and can offer help, advice, and empathy.

Another outlet for finding a therapist is the Worldwide
Web. Therapists who specialize in gut-related issues will
likely have links to IBS sites. You can also visit chat rooms
and put the word out that you're looking for a therapist.
Not only may you get some helpful recommendations, but
you may also be alerted about therapists to avoid.

Be sure to check the licensing of any therapist you consider. A psychologist or psychiatrist must undergo post-
graduate education and an internship with experienced
professionals before receiving credentials. Therapists who
refer to themselves as "counselors" or offer "alternative"
services may not have such a solid background. It's true,
however, that many licensed therapists consider and use alternative methods along with more traditional therapies.
Of course, schooling is no guarantee of skill or profes-
sionalism, but it does offer you one way to review and
consider a therapist's credentials.

Once you've acquired a list of possible therapists, set
up interview appointments. Make a list of questions and
issues that are important to you. Here are some matters
you may want to ask a prospective therapist about:

- Do you have other patients with IBS or similar
  stress-related physical ailments, such as fibromyalgia?
- Have you received any special training or done
  any research in such issues?
- Which specific therapeutic practices have you

used successfully to help others? Do you use cognitive-behavioral techniques?

➤ For what length of time should I expect to continue therapy?

No pun intended, but you should trust your gut reaction to the therapists you interview. If someone makes you feel uncomfortable, don't think you need to analyze or understand why. Simply say thank you and go on to the next interview until you find someone with whom you feel comfortable and safe.

A therapeutic course of treatment is never cut and dried, and the initial impetus—dealing with IBS—may lead you to uncover difficult issues of abuse or trauma that require longer and more intense treatment than you originally planned. However, for many patients, treatment is a fairly concrete process of identifying and coping with stressors, whether external or internal. Look for a therapist who practices this type of practical therapy. The old-fashioned notion of spending twenty years on a couch may make great fodder for Woody Allen movies, but it's probably not the most practical, proactive, or expedient choice for coping with IBS.

Spirituality and Stress Management

Although many people connect spirituality directly to a specific faith, you need not go to a place of worship, or even believe in God, to tap into the peace of connecting to something greater than yourself.

Finding Help in Faith

If you are uncomfortable seeking help from a therapist, or even uncomfortable seeking a therapist to begin with, your place of worship can be a good place to start "talking it out" with a caring professional. Your priest, rabbi, minister, or other religious leader may not have specific experience with the problem of IBS, but he certainly will have had experience dealing with the toll that life's stress takes on the members of a congregation. When you feel embarrassed or ashamed about a problem, you may find a sense of safety in talking to someone who shares your values, knows your family, perhaps even presided at your marriage, bar mitzvah, or christening. A member of the clergy may also know of a traditional therapist who shares your faith and values, with whom you'd be comfortable.

If you are one of the many people who are very hard on themselves, a spiritual counselor may well help you to ease up, to remember that you cannot control—nor are you responsible for—everything and everyone around you. Reconnecting with and strengthening your faith can bring peace, and with it an ability to relax and let go a little of day-to-day irritations and upsets. Individually, they may be minor, but they pile up one by one to take a big toll on your life and health.

For some people, visiting a house of worship—even if it is one that they don't regularly attend or one not of their own religion—provides a real calm. Don't think of a church, synagogue, or mosque as a place you visit only when attending services; it can offer an excellent refuge for peaceful reflection, contemplation, and relaxation.

Personally, I have always loved St. Peter and Paul's Cathedral in my hometown of San Francisco, although I am not Catholic. Whenever I visit the city, I find myself drawn there to think about loved ones both living and dead, to light a candle, to sit quietly in the mostly empty church, and to think about things I've done and things I hope to do. Perhaps the building holds the faith of the many who have been there before, perhaps the architect was divinely inspired—whatever the reason, I always feel better after even the briefest visit there.

Finding the Spiritual in Nature

Not everyone is comfortable with organized religion or believes in God. It is certainly not necessary to be involved with either to have a sense of the spiritual in the world. An excellent place to pursue that link is in nature.

The natural world offers endless opportunities for the stress reduction afforded by exercise. Leisurely walking or vigorous hiking, cross-country skiing, or a swim in a pond—the physical benefits are obvious. However, you also reap the benefits of being away from the stimuli and constant noises of daily life—phones, beepers, blaring music, television, computers, and the rest. You may suddenly find yourself almost overwhelmed by a long-lost phenomenon—the ability to hear your own thoughts!

Whether you are on a deserted beach, in a grove of redwood trees, in the desert during a star-filled night, or in the middle of a backyard vegetable patch, nature has a way of reminding you that you are a small part of a much greater whole—one that was here long before you and will remain long after you leave. You get a sense of perspective, and perspective can greatly diminish stress. It helps you to take a breath and stop dwelling on every little failure and problem—whether real or perceived.

Whenever possible, take a "nature break"—a walk in the woods, a trip to the lake or ocean, even a brief foray into the local park. When that's not possible, bring a little nature to you. Even nurturing a small plant at the office or planting a few flowers or some rosemary in the window box of a city apartment can take you out of yourself for a brief respite and replace a moment of stress or irritation with one of peace.

The joys of nature can also be found in books. Search bookstores—new or used—to find collections of the poems of Walt Whitman and Robert Frost, the photographs of Ansel Adams, the landscape paintings of Pisarro and Monet. Bring home one or two that particularly appeal to you. They can take you momentarily away from the cares of the day to that more peaceful place in the great outdoors.

Finding Help Through Prayer and Meditation

The benefits of prayer and meditation have been understood and recorded throughout history. Most great spiritual leaders went away alone to pursue those very activities. No child goes through Christian Sunday school unaware of Jesus' forty days and nights alone in the desert. Yet there is little detail about what went on during this well-known chapter in his life. What we do know is this:

When it was over, he came back to his people filled with acceptance of whatever his life would bring.

Whether you believe Jesus to be the Son of God, a remarkable mortal, or a creature of myth is not important to learn lessons from his story. First, prayer and meditation should be private—to reveal their details is to remove their power. Second, practiced faithfully and seriously, they can lead to an acceptance of self and life that is very important to people whose stressors are linked to issues of control, self-doubt, and guilt.

Prayer can be traditional, such as a recitation of the Lord's Prayer or the Sabbath ritual of Judaism. It can also be as individual as a momentary talk with God in a church pew or a vacant elevator. The benefits are multiple, and for the IBS sufferer perhaps even more than for others. Prayer involves taking time away from others to deal with issues of self. Prayer is about asking for help and admitting that you can't do, or control, it all. Prayer brings the comforts of ritual and tradition, the comforts of a heritage and faith greater than our own problems, linking us to those who have suffered hardships far greater than our own. Prayer offers perspective.

Meditation is not associated with a particular religious language or practice. It is, simply put, the process of focusing on one particular thing with complete and total concentration. Throughout the centuries, meditation has been used to broaden spiritual awareness, battle addictions and physical ailments, improve the quality of life, and heighten focus and concentration. The earliest writings that record the practice of meditation are found in sacred Hindu texts called the Vedas, which were set down in

India in 1500 B.C. Later, in the sixth century B.C., the Taoists of China, Buddhists of India, and ancient Greeks all practiced some form of meditation.

The focus of meditation can be an object, a mental image, a repeated physical behavior, or a repeated word, phrase, or sound. In Buddhism, a group or individual may induce a meditative state by repeating the phrase *nomniyorengaku*. Others may use a yoga posture to begin the meditative process. When a meditative state is achieved, the physical condition is not unlike that of a person who has been hypnotized. This state brings with it a deep physical and psychic relaxation.

To learn more about the practice of meditation, you can investigate the teachings of Buddhism and yoga, as well as writings by alternative practitioners such as Louise Haye.

It is possible to teach yourself to meditate. You need the following:

- A peaceful location where you won't be interrupted by either people or phones.
- A comfortable position. Some people employ the traditional, cross-legged yoga posture; others simply use a straight-backed chair. Whatever you choose, your spine should be straight and upright.
- A point of focus. This can be your breathing; an image or object such as a flowering plant, a statue or picture of a religious icon; or a repeated word or phrase.

Breath slowly and rhythmically. Focus on your image or phrase, keep your mind from wandering, remain as passive as possible. Over time, the tendency to have random thoughts lessens, and the meditative state is achieved naturally and instinctively.

Try to schedule your sessions for the same time each day. Many people find that starting the day with meditation greatly improves their ability to cope with daily traumas. A brief session at the end of the day may clear your mind and promote calm and restful sleep. During particularly stressful times, incorporating a ten- to fifteen-minute session at the beginning and again at the end of the day may inhibit an increase of IBS symptoms and attacks.

In addition to meditation, many alternative therapies have been shown to offer benefit to IBS sufferers. In chapter seven we'll detail more of these therapies along with studies by traditional medical practitioners who have documented their promise and positive results.

Keeping Stress-Relievers Close at Hand

Although eliminating stress is a long-term project, many immediate, short-term alleviators of stress also offer real benefit. Over the long term, you need to keep examining, identifying, and coping with stressors, altering your lifestyle in terms of diet, exercise, and interactions in relationships. In the short term, you can learn how to get through a stressful moment successfully. You will doubtless find that those moments add up to feeling better a significant amount of the time. The following group of immediate stress-relievers is entirely personal, and some may seem silly, but if nothing else, they may prompt you to think of some objects, writings, or activities that would help you defuse when things get too tense.

Humor

- ✦ *Favorite cartoons.* From Garfield to collections from *The New Yorker,* your favorites probably have been the subject of a calendar or date book. Buy one, and keep it on your desk or in your kitchen. When things get bad, take a moment to flip through and find a laugh.
- ✦ *Great humorous stories.* Most of us have one or two stories—about family, work, or a stranger in a restaurant—that always get a laugh when we tell them. Not only do our listeners laugh, but we too burst into laughter as we tell these tales. Take the time to record them on paper, and keep several copies handy. When you're hit with stress, pull out the paper, read it, and connect with the good feelings aroused by considering both the story and the fun you've had telling it. In those few moments, you can reduce your stress and regain perspective.
- ✦ *An entertaining friend.* Some people always cheer you up, whether with the latest joke or a consistently funny take on a difficult situation. Call your friend for a quick lift.
- ✦ *Comedies on video.* Buy a couple of your favorites to have on hand. Even if you don't always have time to enjoy the entire movie, watching a favorite scene can offer a break and ease a bad mood.

A Return to Childhood

Reincorporating some of your favorite childhood activities into your adult life can help you reconnect to happier or less-complicated times. Try some of the following:

- ➤ *Coloring.* Some adults swear by the benefits of a coloring book for relieving stress. Before you dismiss this out of hand, remember that it doesn't have to be Pokémon! There are many beautiful books depicting the Renaissance, Elizabethan England, Victoriana, and the like. If this idea appeals to you but you're afraid others will think you are silly, remember that not worrying so much about what others think of you is part of the healing process.
- ➤ *Building a fort.* You don't have to construct one out of chairs and blankets the way you used to when you were little, although that might be fun. Do you remember how safe it felt under that canopy? You can make an open-air fort by bringing some of your favorite things— books, tea, journal—onto the couch or bed and shutting out the rest of the world for a while. If your house is usually full, arrange to have your husband take the kids out, or send the kids to stay with a neighbor and let your husband take his own break with friends.
- ➤ *Reading a book from your childhood.* Revisiting the pages of Louisa May Alcott or *The Lion, the Witch, and the Wardrobe* can take you back to the magical discovery of the joys of

reading and offer welcome relief from the gritty sex and violence that fills most of adult reading matter, whether newspapers or fiction.

→ *Playing a game.* Get your kids and some friends together, and pull out the Monopoly board or dust off your skill at charades. There is one caveat to this—if you or any of your fellow players is highly competitive, this activity could actually create stress. If it's not going to be silly and fun, don't do it.

Spiritual Reminders

The most basic elements of spirituality—prayer, meditation, contemplation—can be practiced anywhere there is quiet and privacy. However, carrying small reminders or icons of your faith with you can help you connect with your spirituality in moments of stress.

→ A *favorite prayer, proverb, or poem.* Copy your spiritual reminder, and keep it in your wallet. Pull it out and read it when you feel the need for comfort and calm.

→ *An icon.* Keep a cross, a Star of David, a flower pressed from a favorite hike. Hang it from a necklace or key chain, or tuck it into an easily accessible drawer and reach for it when you feel that clenching in your stomach. It can take you to a calmer, quieter place.

→ A *quiet place.* Maybe it's a courtyard near your office or a quiet side street by your house. Find a place where you can go and be alone, even if only for five minutes, to catch your breath and calm yourself away from ringing phones and demanding co-workers or children.

→ *A nearby bit of nature.* Your miniature oasis doesn't have to be growing if your green thumb leans more to brown. A seashell or collection of pebbles can also be a comforting link to the great outdoors.

→ *A portable photo album.* Think of the favorite photographs that immediately bring a smile to your face. Take four or five to your local copy store and make a page that you can slip into your purse, wallet, backpack, or workspace. That image of your two-year-old covered in spaghetti or a group of friends clowning on a ski slope may be just what you need in an unhappy or overwhelming moment.

→ *Favorite Web sites.* If you spend a lot of time on the computer, "bookmark" sites to get quick and easy access to favorites that offer you a momentary diversion from pressure and stress. The variety available on the Web is endless. For example, while browsing one day, I found a London art gallery that specializes in beautiful early-twentieth-century landscapes and portraits. Whenever I needed a break from the somewhat drab surroundings of that office, I'd click over and spend a minute or two in a 1900s garden. That little bit of beauty offered a lot of relief. Travel sites can offer great diversions. One African wildlife preserve has a twenty-four-hour Web camera recording the comings and goings of lions and water buffalo. Whether you prefer humor, art, travel, or some other subject, the Web offers a wealth of quick stress-relievers.

These are just a few of the many possibilities for relieving stress. My purpose is to get you to think of some new and interesting ways to help yourself when things get rough. Too often we rely on the familiar—plopping down in front of the TV, grabbing a brownie, rehashing problems with a friend—when we're feeling overwhelmed. They may feel good at the moment, but these activities may not offer long-term benefit or real relief from stress. Breaking out of a rut—ceasing to react to stressors in the same old way—can, in and of itself, offer relief.

CHAPTER SEVEN

Alternative Therapies

In recent years Western medicine has become more interested in, and accepting of, Eastern medicine and other nontraditional treatments. Pioneers such as Dr. Andrew Weil have brought alternative medicine into the mainstream, and what may have seemed strange or even frightening to many people twenty years ago is now commonly understood by the average *Oprah* viewer.

Some alternative practices have shown great promise in the treatment of IBS, either by directly relieving symptoms or by aiding relaxation and stress-reduction. Some of the most concrete evidence has been found in a study on the benefits of Chinese herbal medicine.

Chinese Herbal Medicine

The tradition of Chinese herbal medicine (CHM) is more than two thousand years old and is part of the whole system of Chinese medicine. The groundwork for Chinese health practices was established by the great philosopher Lao-tzu, who founded Taoism in the sixth century B.C. In his writings Lao-tzu described the two opposite and complementary forces present in each individual—*yin* and *yang*—and the need to keep them in balance. He introduced the concept of *qi* (pronounced "chee" and sometimes written *chi*), the vital energy force that flows through the body. Blockage of *qi* is believed to cause illness and diminished physical capacity. Chinese medicine is concerned with the individual's complete health, although treatments may address specific symptoms and blockages.

The well-known Western *Journal of the American Medical Association (JAMA)* (November 11, 1998) published the results of a randomized, double-blind study conducted from 1996 to 1997, showing that CHM offered significant benefits to IBS sufferers. The study's 116 patients were randomly given one of three preparations—a general Chinese herbal preparation, an herbal preparation tailored specifically to the symptoms and needs of the patient, or a placebo. Patients were recruited through teaching hospitals and the private practices of gastroenterologists and were given the herbal preparations at one of three Chinese herbal clinics.

The course of treatment lasted sixteen weeks. Each patient was evaluated by a gastroenterologist at the beginning of the study, at eight weeks, and at sixteen weeks. Neither the patients nor the gastroenterologists nor the herbalists were informed which patient received which preparation. (The herbalists were given specifications of symptoms to tailor preparations to, rather than identities of patients with those symptoms.) No other changes were made in the patient's routine, although the study instructions suggested that patients avoid foods they knew would provoke an IBS attack.

At the beginning of the study both patients and their gastroenterologists independently completed the Bowel Symptom Scale, a questionnaire designed to grade patient symptoms and discomfort. They rated the severity and frequency of symptoms—stool passage, cramping, diarrhea, and the like—as well as the degree to which the symptoms of IBS affected the patients' daily lives. They also recorded any adjustments patients had made in their use of medication or consumption of fiber. A brief follow-up questionnaire was administered at two, four, ten, and sixteen weeks. This study model had previously been successful in evaluating the benefits of both various forms of psychological treatment and acupuncture. It has proved both consistent and reliable during retesting.

In five outcome measures, both patients and gastroenterologists assessed frequency and severity of symptoms and interference with daily life. In all five, patients receiving the standard general blend of herbal medicine fared significantly better than those receiving placebos. Those who received an herbal blend tailored to their symptoms fared better than the placebo counterparts in four out of the five measures; although, interestingly, they did not do quite as well as those receiving the more general herbal treatment.

At the end of the trial, 76 percent of patients receiving the standard CHM blend felt that they had improved during treatment, 64 percent of those receiving customized CHM treatment felt that they had, and 32 percent of those receiving placebos felt that they had. It is interesting that simply participating in the study helped some patients. Examinations by gastroenterologists confirmed improvement, although the doctors' assessments of improvement differed somewhat from the patients'. In the physicians' judgments, 78 percent of those receiving general CHM, 50 percent of those receiving individualized CHM, and 30 percent of those taking placebos were better at the end of the study.

Post-study evaluations revealed that for some patients the benefits continued for up to fourteen weeks after treatment ended. Patients who received individualized preparations showed the greatest long-term benefits. Only two subjects opted to leave the study as a result of adverse reactions to the herbs.

If CHM is a treatment you'd like to try, be sure to do some research to find a reputable herbalist. Check the Web for articles listed in the bibliography at the end of this book and other medical articles about treatment with Chinese herbs. Those articles may list research facilities or hospitals in your area that can recommend a reputable practitioner. Many Chinese herbalists are part of a local group or society that is also listed on the Web or in other directories. If you know a good acupuncturist, she can likely lead you to a good herbal practitioner or may herself be a practitioner.

Proceed with caution, and certainly do not attempt self-medication with herbs. Although studies may outline which herbs and quantities were used during a particular trial, buying those herbs in a shop or on-line and attempting to prepare your own dosage could be dangerous. You should no more consider doing that than attempt to prescribe a more traditional Western medicine for yourself.

Acupuncture

Another primary component of Chinese medicine is acupuncture, a therapy that consists of inserting hair-thin needles slightly into the skin at established points throughout the body to restore the balance of *yin* and *yang* and release blocked flows of energy, *qi,* through the body.

Although acupuncture is not accepted here as the cure-all it was believed to be in ancient China, modern Western medicine does recognize it as beneficial in the treatment of pain, nausea, and vomiting, and addiction to drugs and alcohol. For the IBS sufferer, acupuncture can offer documented help in managing pain. Some also find that it aids in stress relief, and lack of definitive proof of such benefits in no way makes them less valid or useful to individuals.

There are several ways to find a reputable acupuncturist. First, more and more Western doctors are discovering that acupuncture can offer their patients pain relief, so your general practitioner or gastroenterologist may have a recommendation for you. Alternatively, consult national professional associations such as the American Association of Acupuncture and Oriental Medicine or the National Commission for the Certification of Acupuncturists. Also check your local library, directory assistance, or the Worldwide Web for complete listings of acupuncture practitioners.

Biofeedback

Physicians and researchers are increasingly accepting of, and working to understand, the mind/body connection. Biofeedback is one concrete way of measuring the physical reactions caused by various stressors. It enables patients first to identify and subsequently to anticipate and counter the stressors with techniques designed to promote calm and relaxation and to inhibit stress-provoked symptoms.

Biofeedback uses monitoring equipment to register physical reactions to outside stimuli. The reactions can be viewed on a computer screen. Different methods of biofeedback are used to monitor and address different conditions.

- *Electromyography (EMG)* measures muscle tension and treats muscle pain, chronic stiffness, and incontinence. It is also a useful tool for rehabilitation of injured muscles.
- *Thermal biofeedback* measures skin temperature, which indicates changes in blood flow. It can be used to relieve hypertension, migraines, anxiety, and Raynaud's disease (a periodic loss of circulation in fingers or toes or both that results in abnormal coldness in those extremities).
- *Electrodermal activity (EDA) sensors* measure otherwise undetectable changes in perspiration and are frequently used in the treatment of anxiety.
- *Galvanic skin response (GSR) sensors* track the amount of perspiration produced during stressful situations as a measure of skin conductivity. These sensors are used to reduce anxiety.
- *Finger pulse feedback* measures both the pulse rate and the amount of blood in each pulse. These measurements can help patients control hypertension, anxiety, and cardiac arrhythmias.

➤ *Electrocardiographs* track heart rate and can assist in the treatment of excessively rapid heartbeat and in the control of high blood pressure.

➤ *Electroencephalographs* are used to measure brain activity. Conditions that are potentially treatable by this feedback include attention deficit disorder (ADD), depression, hyperactivity, and tooth-grinding.

Once patients' physiologic responses have been identified, biofeedback training enables the patients to gain control over their responses. The responses normally should be unconscious and automatic, but they are malfunctioning and thus producing a variety of unpleasant symptoms, such as chronic pain, insomnia, fatigue, and hypertension. Biofeedback has been successful in treating disorders ranging from alcoholism to attention deficit disorder, high blood pressure, and abnormal heart rates. Most significantly for the purposes of this book, they have treated digestive disorders including IBS.

Biofeedback is not a passive treatment or a quick fix; it requires commitment, focus, and dedication by patients. It consists of the daunting task of controlling functions that are easy and automatic when patients are healthy but seem frighteningly out of control when the body isn't functioning as it should.

After you answer standard questions about your own health and your family's health history, a biofeedback technician will attach sensors to your body in accordance with the areas that require treatment. If you have tension and heart problems, sensors are attached to the skin; for migraines and depression, devices are used on the scalp;

for Raynaud's disease, the fingers and toes are monitored; and so on.

Sensors indicate where and when improper involuntary responses happen, and then a therapist instructs you in mental or physical exercises that affect the functional disorder. By watching the screen, you see how these exercises positively affect your reactions, and with time and patience you learn to control and correct the physiologic problem. In general, eight to ten sessions of thirty minutes to an hour, occurring from one to five times a week, are sufficient for you to learn the techniques and reap the benefits. Some more complex syndromes, such as ADD, may require as many as forty sessions. Patient commitment and focus are factors in the length and success of treatment.

Unlike other alternative practices, biofeedback does not address whole body wellness or general health. Rather, it addresses the need to control and alter specific problem-causing responses. The benefits to the IBS sufferer are clear—not only can biofeedback address specific physical symptoms, but it can also help break the vicious cycle of stress that provokes symptoms that create more stress.

Be sure to choose a biofeedback practitioner who has have been certified by the Biofeedback Certification Institute of America. Most major cities have biofeedback associations, or your doctor or local hospital may have a recommendation for you. The Worldwide Web is a good place to find referrals and to check credentials.

Hypnosis

While doing research on the Web, I came upon a number of personal Web sites posted by IBS sufferers who had experienced significant benefits from hypnotherapy. Researchers are also increasingly hopeful about the potential benefits of this therapy for IBS. Indeed, as early as 1989 the British medical journal *Lancet* reported that half of forty IBS subjects treated with hypnotherapy over a seven-week period enjoyed improved health, and eleven of those became almost symptom-free. Their improvements lasted for three months after the therapy was finished.

Hypnosis is an ancient practice that in its earliest incarnations was a component of both magic and religion. Native Americans used hypnosis in healing rites, inducing the hypnotic state through chanting or, on occasion, the use of hallucinogenic drugs.

The modern medical uses of hypnosis were introduced by the Viennese physician Franz Mesmer (hence the verb to *mesmerize*). Like the Chinese, Mesmer believed that illness was the result of a body out of balance, although he thought that the imbalances occurred in what he termed the body's natural "animal magnetism." They could be righted by using calming words and gestures that induced relaxation and promoted wellness. Although the specifics of his theories did not gain much of a following, the general notion of incorporating alteration of consciousness with standard medical treatment did gain acceptance.

Hypnosis has been extraordinarily successful in reducing all types of pain. It has even been used effectively in place of anesthetics in surgery for patients who cannot tolerate drugs. Hypnotherapy has relieved psychological conditions such as anxiety, depression, compulsions, and phobias and may be used to treat a variety of addictions.

Hypnotherapy doesn't cure disease, but it does offer great relief from many debilitating symptoms in conditions as common as allergies and as serious as Parkinson's disease. It can alleviate side effects of medical treatment, such as nausea from chemotherapy or excessive bleeding from surgery. Pregnant women who are suffering extreme morning sickness may find safe and prompt relief through hypnotherapy. While as many as 90 percent of the population can be hypnotized, it does not, unfortunately, work for everyone. Some people are simply not good candidates for the procedure.

If you want to try hypnotherapy, the first session will focus on just that question: Are you a good candidate for hypnosis? A variety of tests can indicate to a trained hypnotherapist whether you are likely to be hypnotized or not.

- *The Stanford Hypnotic Susceptibility Scales* encompass twelve exercises of increasing difficulty. The first entails simply closing your eyes and falling forward or backward; the last involves your response to "posthypnotic suggestion." In such a test, the hypnotist might instruct you to get up and open and close the door, or take a drink of water, each time he snaps his fingers. Most people are successful in the first exercise, but few can complete all twelve. The more exercises you complete, the greater the likelihood that you can be hypnotized.
- *The Barber Suggestibility Scale* is an eight-task test, similar in nature to the Stanford Scales. Again, you are encouraged to respond to stimuli—perhaps to scratch your nose each time the hypnotist taps her pencil on the desk, or to imagine that you cannot lift your leg. The more

tests you complete successfully, the better your chances of being hypnotized.

→ *The Harvard Group Scale of Hypnotic Susceptibility* also has twelve exercises, but it is given to a group and as a result is not considered as reliable as the others.

Other, less complex and therefore less reliable, tests include

→ *Eye rolling,* in which you open the eye wide, roll the eye up, and then attempt to lower the lid while the eye is in the upward position.

→ *The light test,* in which you stare at a spot of light on the wall in a darkened room. If you perceive that it not only moves but also frequently changes direction, you are supposed to be susceptible to hypnosis.

→ *The lemon test* in which you imagine holding, slicing, and juicing a lemon. If this induces conscious salivation, hypnosis may be successful.

Common techniques to induce hypnosis include the classic focusing on a moving object as it swings back and forth; focusing on the sound of the therapist's voice as she gives a series of instructions; and counting backward from thirty. (Who has never seen a movie or television show in which a man swings a pocket watch by its chain in front of a subject and announces, "You are getting sleepy, very sleepy"? It may be a cliché, but it works.)

In a hypnotic trance state, you experience deep relaxation. The outer world becomes less concrete and your focus turns to your own emotions and sensations. You no longer control your thoughts and emotions as you do in a conscious state. The therapist will instruct you to focus on peaceful imagery, such as a stroll on the beach or observing stars on a clear summer night.

Once you have cleared your mind of painful or unpleasant thoughts, the therapist will make suggestions designed to alleviate or eliminate your pain or other symptoms. She may help you address conscious memories or emotions that could be linked to your condition. Posthypnotic suggestions may be offered to help you continue to deal with problems or symptoms after the session is finished. The therapist may tell a smoker, for example, that the smell of smoke will induce nausea. The therapist then generally suggests that you will feel well and relaxed upon waking, and she brings you out of the trance.

The potential for IBS relief is clear. Perhaps your gut always reacts when you are about to attend a social occasion because you are anxious about having an IBS attack in an unfamiliar place. A therapist might offer the suggestion that socializing relaxes you. Hypnosis can address both specific symptoms (as biofeedback does) and general health by relieving stress and anxiety.

Once you have attended a few sessions, the hypnotherapist will likely instruct you in the art of self-hypnosis. A variety of tapes purport to teach people to hypnotize themselves without the assistance of a trained therapist; but there is no way to vouch for their efficacy, let alone to self-test your susceptibility to hypnosis.

Almost anyone can practice hypnotherapy without breaking the law, but you don't want to trust your subconscious to just anyone or waste your time and money on quacks. Seek out an accredited psychiatrist or psychotherapist who has extensive experience with both hypnotherapy and your particular complaint.

A number of reputable associations of hypnotists can be located in the local yellow pages, through national directory assistance, or on the Web. They include the American Institute of Hypnotherapy in Santa Ana, California, and the National Guild of Hypnotists in Merrimack, New Hampshire.

Don't be shy about asking your physician for a referral to a hypnotist. The medical benefits of this therapy are widely accepted. You might also try the anesthesiology department of your local hospital, which may use the services of a hypnotist for patients who are intolerant of anesthetics.

Creative Visualization

The technique of creative visualization was introduced to millions of people in the book of the same name by Shakti Gawain. The book addresses the concept of envisioning what you want for yourself—be it a prosperous career, love, or good health. For the IBS sufferer, the focus will be on health and relaxation. It is not necessary to have a picture in your mind but rather to focus on an idea or goal.

One of the techniques of visualization is to create a daily affirmation page in your journal. There you write your desire over and over again. For instance, you might fill a page with the sentence "Food brings pleasure and relaxation" or "I am relaxed and happy in my work" or perhaps "I am doing good when I take care of myself."

Affirmations can also be used to help you maintain healthy habits. For instance, you might regularly affirm to yourself that you love healthy food or are excited and happy to take a brief walk and meditate each morning. Driving out the negative (I hate to exercise) with positive self-messages can be a very useful and beneficial process.

Affirmations can also help when the problem that's bothering you is another person. Pick one or two positive attributes of the person who is causing you stress or with whom you frequently clash. Repeat these positive thoughts about the person to yourself as often as possible, and take a moment to write them down. Not always, but often, the more positive energy you inevitably send out to that person will improve the relations between you. I'm not saying that you'll become best friends (although odder things have happened), but time together should become much more tolerable.

All these therapies offer a positive, proactive way to deal with your IBS symptoms. Remember that it's important to do your research and find a reputable practitioner. And you need to be well informed about the therapies you're considering so that you ask the right questions to find the correct specialist and treatment for you.

CHAPTER EIGHT

Medication Strategies

D
rug therapies for IBS became headline news in 2000 with the fast-track approval of the IBS drug Lotronex and its subsequent ban and removal from the market. One positive effect of this unfortunate and harmful episode is that more people are aware of IBS, and many sufferers now know that they are not alone. However, the complications, some potentially fatal, that resulted from taking Lotronex vividly illustrate the dangers of fast-track approval of drugs.

The Lotronex Fiasco

Lotronex was specifically targeted to women whose primary IBS symptom was diarrhea. It was made available on February 9, 2000, and by November 2000 the FDA had received ninety-three reports of patients hospitalized after taking Lotronex, forty-nine of whom developed ischemic colitis, a potentially lethal complication resulting from inadequate blood flow to the colon. At the end of that month the FDA requested the drug's manufacturer, Glaxo Wellcome, to remove Lotronex from the market, although Glaxo maintains that it is safe and efficacious.

A report by the *Los Angeles Times* (November 2, 2000) showed that the FDA had been remiss in its approval of Lotronex. The *Times* investigation revealed that the FDA

- Ignored significant concerns raised by a doctor within the FDA who had considered Lotronex before its approval
- Included a paid consultant for Glaxo on the advisory committee that approved the drug
- Granted Glaxo's request not to require a highly visible "black box" warning on the Lotronex label
- Approved Lotronex with the condition that Glaxo would conduct a major study on potential links between the drug and ischemic colitis, rather than waiting to approve the drug until that study was concluded (when Lotronex was removed from the market, the study still had not begun)

As awareness of IBS continues to grow, there is no doubt that drug companies—well aware of a potentially profitable market—will be racing to find a cure, or at least a pharmaceutical aid, for the syndrome. Although medicine is the best treatment in some instances, it often is not in others. Still, many IBS patients show a marked preference for the "simple" choice of a pill over more proactive behavior.

Think of the person with Type II diabetes who prefers medicine to losing the twenty pounds that might make drug treatment unnecessary. Consider the readiness with which some psychiatrists—often spurred by HMOs—dispense pills instead of engaging their patients in talk therapy.

This is not to say that medicine can't help. It can. But new therapies should be approached cautiously and old ones used judiciously. Avoid the potential quick fix that could leave you worse off than you were before.

That said, *Reuters Health* (November 28, 2000) reported that a Swiss pharmaceutical group, Novartis, has completed the data necessary to receive marketing approval for the IBS drug Zelmac (tegaserod) sometime in 2001 and also hopes to have it approved in Europe at that time.

Croton lechleri:
A Supplemental Option

In the Amazon and other tropical regions of South America there grows a tree commonly known as *sangre de drago* (blood of the dragon), so named because the tree emits a dark red sap when it is cut or damaged. For centuries, indigenous people of South America have used this sap, as well as preparations made from the tree's bark, in a variety of fashions. When painted on an injury, the sap forms a seal that stops bleeding, promotes healing, and offers protection from injury and infection. The sap is also used to treat mouth ulcers and (of primary interest to IBS sufferers) diarrhea.

Sangre de grado is a tree of the genus *Croton,* which has a number of species, including *Croton lechleri.* Legal and approved for use in the United States, *Croton* has not been publicized until recently, because studies of the plant have been done primarily by pharmaceutical companies seeking to create patented medicines or supplements from it. Shaman Botanicals, of South San Francisco, California, was preparing in 2001 to introduce an antidiarrheal supplement created from *Croton lechleri* resin. Other researchers are pursuing the plant's healing properties as an anti-inflammatory, pain reliever, and wound treatment.

An agent isolated from the *Croton lechleri* tree, Provir (also called SP-303), has undergone experimental trials. In double-blind studies presented at the Thirty-sixth Annual Meeting of the Infectious Diseases Society of America, 184 travelers to Mexico and Jamaica who suffered acute diarrhea were given either Provir or a placebo. Those receiving a 250 mg dose of Provir showed marked improvement: over 90 percent experienced partial or complete improvement within twenty-four hours.

A study performed jointly by the University of North Carolina at Chapel Hill and Shaman Botanicals examined the effects of SP-303 on mice with cholera-toxin–induced diarrhea. The *Croton* drug reduced the excess fluid in the intestine associated with this extremely watery diarrhea and so promoted relief of the condition and formation of normal stools.

Croton works differently from other antidiarrheals. Loperamide products, such as Imodium, inhibit diarrhea by reducing intestinal motility; because of this they may cause constipation. Psyllium products, such as Metamucil, bulk stools effectively but have to be taken frequently, which some users find unpleasant. *Croton* is a promising alternative.

It's important to consult your doctor and proceed cautiously when trying this supplement, like all new products. Both *Croton*-based supplements and *Croton lecheri* in its natural form can be purchased in health food stores and on Web sites. Before using any unfamiliar product, be sure you receive professional instruction from a reputable doctor, nutritionist, or herbalist about your course of treatment. "Natural" is no guarantee of safety or efficacy.

Zelmac and Women with IBS

Researchers have said that Zelmac is intrinsically safer than Lotronex. Zelmac is designed for women whose predominant symptom is constipation rather than diarrhea. A placebo-controlled study of 799 patients showed that a daily dose of the drug relieved abdominal pain from the second day of treatment. Bloating decreased during the first week, and bowel function improved from the first day. Because relief is rapid, patients are more likely to follow the regimen and enjoy long-term benefit. Although not geared toward diarrhea-predominant patients, Zelmac gives no indication that it may harm them, and, because most IBS sufferers experience at least occasional bouts of diarrhea, it offers some benefit for all female sufferers. Zelmac has shown no noticeable benefit for male IBS patients, and researchers are unclear why the benefits apply only to women.

Antidepressants

Perhaps the most common prescription for IBS sufferers is antidepressants. Although they certainly assist patients who suffer depression in conjunction with an IBS diagnosis, depression need not be present for them to be useful.

Antidepressants also have a documented benefit as pain relievers. A study in the *British Medical Journal* (March 15, 1997) focused on the use of antidepressants to relieve neuropathic pain, atypical facial pain, fibromyalgia, and IBS. When used for analgesic effects, these drugs lessen pain more quickly than they relieve depression, and a smaller dosage is typically required. Antidepressants can act alone in treating functional disorders or as an adjunct to other painkillers in treating chronic conditions such as cancer.

Antidepressants work in IBS by increasing the release of neurotransmitters. These brain chemicals cause signals to be sent down the inhibitory pathway, effectively shutting off the transmission of pain signals from the gut to the brain via the spinal cord.

One of two categories of antidepressants is generally prescribed for pain management:

1. *Tricyclic antidepressants (TCAs)* have been thoroughly studied for their efficacy in pain management and can diminish anxiety and promote deep sleep as well. Elavil is a commonly prescribed TCA. Like all prescription medications, TCAs can have side effects. Common problems include dry mouth, weight gain, and sexual dysfunction. The most dangerous potential side effect is aggravation of heart rhythm disturbances. Cessa-

tion of TCAs may also cause side effects and should be done slowly to avoid GI upset, sleeplessness, nausea, and nightmares, among other possible problems. With all drugs, be sure to follow your doctor's orders to the letter and report any side effects immediately.

2. *Selective serotonin reuptake inhibitors (SSRIs)* are a newer class of antidepressants whose brand names are familiar to most of us, whether we're taking them or not—Effexor, Paxil, Prozac, and Zoloft are all SSRIs. These drugs are best taken at bedtime to minimize side effects, which may include headache and sexual dysfunction. Each patient is affected differently, and each SSRI has side effects specific to it. Some may cause sleeplessness, and those should be avoided by IBS patients who have sleep-deprivation problems. Some SSRIs can cause loose stools, which might actually be beneficial to IBS patients who suffer chronic constipation but could be disastrous for those who suffer cramping and diarrhea. Clearly it's vital to have a detailed discussion with your physician about possible side effects of any drug prescribed for you. Be sure to give the doctor a precise and complete description of all symptoms you have suffered related to IBS or any other condition.

Antibiotics

An interesting study published in the *American Journal of Gastroenterology* (December 2000) suggests that IBS in some patients may be linked to overabundant bacterial growth in the small intestine, which can be successfully treated with antibiotics.

The study looked at 202 subjects who had been diagnosed with IBS using the Rome criteria. They were given a lactulose hydrogen breath test to determine whether they were suffering from an overgrowth of bacteria in the small intestine, and 157 (78 percent of the subjects) were found to have the overgrowth. After a ten-day course of antibiotics, forty-seven of the patients were tested again. Twenty-five had eradicated the bacteria of their small intestine, and 48 percent of those patients no longer met the Rome criteria for IBS. All patients who eradicated the bacteria showed improvement over those who had not.

It may well be worthwhile to bring this study to your physician's attention. Although it obviously does not offer a cure for all IBS patients, it may help some, and one of them may be you.

Antispasmodics

If you suffer from extremely painful and debilitating episodes of cramping and spasm, periodic use of antispasmodic (anticholinergic) drugs may be beneficial. These medicines temporarily block nerve impulses to the muscles of the gut, thereby reducing painful colon spasms. Although the drugs may offer relief from the immediate cramping associated with constipation, if used consistently they can actually promote constipation by inhibiting the spasms and contractions required for proper waste motility.

Antidiarrheals

Antidiarrhea medicines can control and minimize chronic diarrhea. Two common prescriptions are loperamide hydrochloride and diphenoxylate hydrochloride. Loperamide is available in nonprescription form as Imodium A-D and has been shown to actually strengthen the sphincter muscle. It has the added advantage of not entering the brain, which its less-expensive counterpart diphenoxylate does do.

Over-the-Counter Medications

When constipation is an issue, individuals grappling with IBS may overuse laxatives. Stimulant laxatives, including those classified as "all natural," can cause long-term problems, even damage to the large intestine. Although they may offer some immediate relief, over the long term they cause many more problems than they solve. Gentle, non-stimulant bulking agents, such as high-fiber Citrucel, can bring relief and provide an easy solution for IBS patients who need to increase their fiber intake.

Similarly, occasional use of antidiarrheal medicines such as Pepto-Bismol or Kaopectate are fine for dealing with particularly severe attacks but should not be considered a long-term solution.

Antacids such as Pepcid and gas-reducing medications such as Beano have not been evaluated for their efficacy in treating IBS, although anecdotal reports indicate that they may relieve flatulence and cramping. For some, Beano may inhibit the onset of some gas-related symptoms.

If you are taking medication, whether prescribed or over the counter, for any other condition, consider whether potential side effects of that drug may be exacerbating your IBS. Talk to your doctor, and do research on your own.

Many Web sites offer miracle relief for IBS. Often these are herbal treatments touted as all natural, and natural they may be. Opium in its pure form is all natural, as are a variety of potentially dangerous herbs. Herbal therapies can be wonderful, but go to an herbalist or nutritionist to make sure that you get the safest and most efficacious mix possible.

Epilogue

NOW THAT YOU HAVE FINISHED reading this book, it's time to put these techniques to use. To do so effectively, think of yourself as your own primary physician or caretaker.

Go through the book again, marking and listing those sections that best apply to you. Then create a manageable game plan for yourself.

Consider which recommendations for your condition seem easiest to tackle and which seem hardest. Perhaps keeping a diet diary sounds interesting or challenging, but learning to say no to others seems overwhelming. Tackle the easy ones first—success breeds success. The more you feel in control of your life, the more you'll be able to take even more control.

Include your family and friends in the process of getting well by letting them know what you're going through, rather than isolating yourself because of a misplaced sense of shame or embarrassment. You have nothing to be embarrassed about. Rather than skipping an evening out or a family party, simply inform friends and relatives that you're having some stress-related stomach problems. There's no need to go into details if you don't want to, but let them know that you may be making a number of trips to the bathroom. Assure them that the problem is not serious, that you don't want them to make a fuss or issue about it, and that if you do have a serious medical emergency, they'll be the first to know! Don't be surprised if alleviating your anxiety about needing to explain results in fewer and less severe symptoms than you had in a previous similar situation.

Learn to love food again. Don't be bound by the conventions about what to eat when. If you made a stew that tastes great to you and you want to eat it for breakfast, lunch, and dinner three days running, go ahead (just don't expect the family to join you). If all you want for dinner is a triple helping of mashed potatoes, fine. Find ways to make mealtimes festive and appealing. Check yard sales for beautiful antique plates; take your dinner outside on an unexpectedly warm night. If a friend makes a dish you truly love, ask her to cook it for you. Go ahead. You'd do it for her.

Create a "time bank." As you chart your progress and begin to notice your symptoms diminishing, you'll find that you have free time that you used to spend coping with your syndrome. As best you can, keep a count of that newly available time. Don't put it all back into chores or things you should do. Save some for enjoying yourself. Go to a movie in the middle of the week. Leave the house early to take yourself out to a quiet breakfast. Play hooky from the Saturday chores to take the kids to the zoo. Let yourself really enjoy feeling good, and reward yourself for the hard work you've done to get better.

Stay informed. At your local library, spend an hour each month or two checking on the latest advances in IBS treatment. If something sounds helpful to you, ask your doctor about it.

Try something new. Do not simply replace your old rut with a new one, falling again into the trap of eating the same foods and doing the same exercises or other stress-relievers. Finding fresh, new ways to take charge of your life and symptoms is empowering and stimulating.

Accept the fact that some days will be better than others. You may be feeling great for days and then, *wham,* an attack hits. Don't be discouraged, and most particularly don't lose perspective. Everybody, including those who don't suffer from IBS, experiences occasional GI problems. Don't overreact to your symptoms. Nobody's life is pain-free; and, no matter how hard you work toward that goal, yours won't be either.

Of course, if, after a period of improvement, your symptoms begin to recur frequently, address that reality. You may need to make new diet and stress diaries. Perhaps you've been neglecting your diet or relaxation techniques without even realizing it. Don't take a flare-up of IBS as a reason to beat yourself up but rather as an opportunity to reevaluate and move forward.

For many people, improving life with IBS is an ongoing, long-term proposition. That doesn't mean it has to be a dreary one. And the care you're taking of yourself to manage IBS has a number of other health benefits, both mental and physical. The attention you're paying to diet and exercise will likely pay off in both an improved figure and a happier outlook. Learning new skills and finding new diversions make you a more interesting and interested person. Perhaps the most valuable benefit can be reconnecting to your own spirituality and the invaluable peace that can bring.

When all is said and done, the once-overwhelming task of coping with your IBS just might—if you let it—

metamorphose into a constructive experience that unexpectedly and positively affects all aspects of your life.

As you gain more and more control of your IBS, it will cease to be the focus of your life and simply become a factor in it. Along the way you will doubtless learn skills that help you in every other aspect of your life—relationships with friends and family, work, and the creative pursuits that are simply for you.

You *can* feel and live better with IBS, and you will—starting right now.

Further Resources

Acupuncture

American Association of Acupuncture and Oriental
  Medicine
433 Front Street
Catasaugua, PA 18032
610-226-1433

National Acupuncture and Oriental Medicine Alliance
  (NAOMA)
www.acuall.org
253-851-6896

American Academy of Medical Acupuncture (AAMA)
1-800-521-2262

Biofeedback

Center for Applied Psychophysiology
Menninger Clinic
PO Box 829
Topeka, KS 66601-0829
913-273-7500, ext. 5375

Society for the Study of Neuronal Regulation (SSNR)
Suite 301
4600 Post Oak Place
Houston TX 77027
713-552-0091

Fibromyalgia

Fibromyalgia Alliance of America, Inc.
PO Box 21990
Columbus, OH 43221-0990
614-457-4222

Fibromyalgia Network
PO Box 31750
Tucson, AZ 85751-1750
520-290-5508
http://alt.med.fibromyalgia

Gastroenterology Referrals

International Foundation for Functional Gastrointestinal
    Disorders
1-888-964-2001

Hypnotherapy

American Council of Hypnotist Examiners
117 East Broadway, Suite 340
Glendale, CA 91205
818-242-5378

National Guild of Hypnotists
PO Box 308
Merrimack, NH 03054
603-429-9438

Meditation

Siddha Yoga Meditation Center
South Fallsburg, NY 12779
918-434-2000

Maharishi Vedic Universities
1-800-434-2000

Tai Chi Chuan

East-West Academy of the Healing Arts
450 Sutter Street, Suite 916
San Francisco, CA 94108
415-788-2227

American Association of Acupuncture and Oriental
    Medicine
433 Front Street
Catasaugua, PA 18032
610-226-1433

Yoga

International Association of Yoga Therapists
109 Hillside Avenue
Mill Valley, CA 94942

American Yoga Association
513 South Orange Avenue
Sarasota, FL 34236
813-953-5859

Glossary

Acupuncture: a primary component of Chinese medicine in which a practitioner inserts hair-thin needles just slightly into the patient's skin at strategic points to promote health and well-being.

Antispasmodics (anticholinergics): medicines that temporarily block nerve impulses to the muscles of the gut, thereby reducing painful colon spasms.

Bacterial gastroenteritis: acute abdominal pain, vomiting, and diarrhea that result from eating or drinking contaminated food or water.

Biofeedback: a treatment that uses electrical sensors and computers to help a patient identify and control stress reactions.

Bipolar disorder (manic-depressive illness): a mental condition that involves a cycle of extreme mood swings from the lows of depression to euphoric highs.

Catastrophizing: self-inducing stress by creating a downward spiral of thoughts that escalate a difficult situation.

Chronic: occurring regularly over an extended period; usually used to describe a symptom or condition.

Chyme: the substance formed in the early stages of digestion when food is broken down and combined with gastric secretions in the stomach.

Cognitive therapy: psychological treatment, individually or in a group, designed to teach the patient to replace negative self-messages with positive ones in order to reduce stress.

Colon: see Large intestine.

Constipation: inhibited bowel movement; the definition can vary from person to person depending on individual bowel motility patterns. For some it means an absence of bowel movement for several days to a week; for others simply difficulty achieving bowel movement.

Conversion syndrome: a syndrome of psychological stress that manifests in a physical way.

Diarrhea: regular passage of soft and watery stools.

Diverticulitis: inflammation of the *diverticula*, which are abnormal pouches that form within the intestinal wall.

Duodenum: the first section of the small intestine, which initially receives chyme from the stomach.

Dysthymia: a chronic form of depression in which the sufferer experiences the symptoms of major depression for more than two years but in a milder form.

Fibromyalgia: a functional disorder characterized by widespread pain in the muscles, tendons, fibrous tissues, and connective tissues and chronic fatigue.

Flatulence: rectal release of excess gas that has formed in the intestinal tract as a result of swallowing air or eating foods that contain undigestible carbohydrate, such as beans.

Functional disorder: a condition that is diagnosed by symptoms rather than the identification of a specific physical cause.

Genus: a natural history or biology class or group with similar attributes; genus is a narrower category than family and a broader category than species.

Globus hystericus: a physical reaction to anxiety or stress that produces the sensation of having a lump in the throat although none is actually present.

Hypnosis: the process of inducing a deeply relaxed state of mind that can be used for a variety of therapeutic purposes.

Ileum: the final section of the small intestine, which absorbs water, fat, bile, and salt before passing digested material into the large intestine.

Inflammatory bowel disease (IBD): A chronic, often debilitating inflammation of the gastric tract.

Irritable bowel syndrome (IBS): a functional disorder characterized by extreme bouts of diarrhea, constipation, cramping, and flatulence, which are triggered primarily by stress and diet.

Jejunum: The middle section of the small intestine, which absorbs carbohydrate and protein from digested material.

Large intestine (colon): the lower part of the digestive tract, which moves waste from the small intestine to its elimination through the anus.

Manic-depressive illness: see Bipolar disorder.

Manning criteria: one of the commonly used sets of criteria by which doctors make an IBS diagnosis.

Motility: the ability of the large intestine to pass waste through so that it can exit the body; increased motility is characterized by diarrhea, decreased motility by constipation.

Nonulcer dyspepsia: a disorder characterized by recurrent or chronic pain in the upper abdomen.

Psychodynamic therapy: one-on-one treatment with a therapist to uncover unconscious triggers of a variety of conditions, including IBS.

Rome criteria: one of the commonly used sets of criteria by which doctors make an IBS diagnosis.

Selective serotonin reuptake inhibitors (SSRIs): the most recently developed class of antidepressants that are sometimes used to reduce pain in the treatment of IBS. They are available in a variety of chemical structures, so one SSRI may work for a particular patient and another may not. Commonly known brand names are Paxil and Zoloft. SSRIs have been shown to produce fewer side effects than tricyclic antidepressants (TCAs), an older class of antidepressants.

Self-blame: a tendency to constantly criticize oneself and take the blame for everything that may go wrong around one.

Self-silencing: the attempt to keep a relationship secure and intact by refraining from expressing actions, feelings, and thoughts that may upset or anger the other person in the relationship.

Sigmoid colon: The lowest section of the large intestine, which empties waste into the rectum.

Species: a natural history or biology group with similar attributes; species is a narrower category than genus, and each species is listed with its genus; some species are further divided into subspecies or varieties.

Stomach: A sacklike organ in the digestive tract that rests beneath the diaphragm and under the rib cage; its primary function is to hold food after ingestion and prepare it for digestion and absorption.

Tricyclic antidepressants (TCAs): a class of antidepressants used for pain management, reduction of anxiety, and promotion of deep sleep in the treatment of IBS. Studied since the 1960s, TCAs are less expensive but more likely to induce side effects than newer antidepressants generally categorized as selective serotonin reuptake inhibitors (SSRIs).

Bibliography

American College of Rheumatology. "1990 Criteria for the Classification of Fibromyalgia." www.co-cure.org. October 6, 1999.

American Gastroenterological Association. Medical Position Statement: "Irritable Bowel Syndrome." Official recommendations approved November 10, 1996.

Bensoussan, A., N. J. Talley, M. Hing, R. Menzies, A. Guo, and M. Ngu. "Treatment of Irritable Bowel Syndrome with Chinese Herbal Medicine: A Randomized Controlled Trial." *Journal of the American Medical Association* 280 (November 11, 1998): 1585.

"Biographical Sketch: Hans Selye." www.heiml.tu-claus thal.de/~heike/selye.shtml

Brostoff, Jonathon, M.D., and Linda Gamlin. *Food Allergies and Food Intolerance*. Rochester, Ver.: Healing Arts Press, 1989.

Carlson, Elizabeth, M.S.N./M.P.H., R.N., A.N.P. "Irritable Bowel Syndrome." *Nurse Practitioner,* January 1998, reproduced on SpringNet–CE Connection. http.//www.springnet.com/celj801a.htm.

Case, A. M., and R. L. Reid. "Effects of the Menstrual Cycle on Medical Disorders." *Archives of Internal Medicine* 158 (July 13, 1998): 1405.

Cassileth, Barrie R., Ph.D. *The Alternative Medicine Handbook*. New York: W. W. Norton & Co., 1998.

Castro, Miranda. *The Homeopathic Guide to Stress*. New York: St. Martin's Griffin, 1996.

Cerda, J. J., and D. A. Drossman. "Effective, Compassionate Management of IBS." *Patient Care* 30 (January 15, 1996): 131.

"Coping with Depression." www.depression.com. May 2000.

"Dear Psych Doc Q&A—Globus Hystericus." http://thriveonline.com.

"Depression—Information and Treatment." www.psychologyinfo.com.

Dicesare, D., H. L. Dupont, J. J. Mathewson, C. D. Ericsson, D. Ashley, F. G. Martinez-Sandoval, J. E. Pennington, and S. B. Porter. "A Double-Blind, Randomized, Placebo-Controlled Study of S-303 (Provir™) in the Symptomatic Treatment of Acute Diarrhea Among Travelers to Mexico and Jamaica." Abstract presented at the Thirty-sixth Annual Meeting of the Infectious Disease Society of America, Denver, 1998.

Drossman, D. A., W. E. Whitehead, and M. Camilleri. "Irritable Bowel Syndrome: A Technical Review for Practice Guideline Development." *Gastroenterology* 112 (1997): 2120–2137.

Estronaut Women's Health Forum. "Irritable Bowel Syndrome in Women." www.estronaut.com.

Falkiewicz, Bogdan, and Jerzy Lukasiak. "Sangre de Drago." Scientific Research. www.HerbSecret.co.UK.

Farthing, Michael J. G. "Irritable Bowel, Irritable Body, or Irritable Brain?" *British Medical Journal* 310 (January 21, 1995): 171.

Gabriel, S. E., S. E. Davenport, R. J. Steagall, V. Vimal, T. Carlson, and E. J. Rozhon. "A Novel Plant-Derived Inhibitor of cAMP-Mediated Fluid and Chloride Secretion." *American Journal of Physiology* 276 (1999): G58-G63.

Gawain, Shakti. *Creative Visualization.* New York: Bantam New Age, 1978.

"Globus Hystericus FAQ." http://www.surgery.ucsd.edu.

Goldberg, Stephen, M.D. *Clinical Anatomy Made Ridiculously Simple.* Miami: Medmaster Inc., 1984.

Gwee, K. A., J. C. Graham, M. W. McKendrick, S. M. Collins, J. S. Marshall, S. J. Walters, and N. W. Read. "Psychometric Scores and Persistence of Irritable Bowel after Infectious Diarrhea." *Lancet* 347 (January 20, 1996): 504.

Harvey, R. F., R. A. Hinton, R. M. Gunary, and R. E. Barry. "Individual and Group Hypnotherapy in Treatment of Refractory Bowel Syndrome." *Lancet* 1 (8653) (February 25, 1989): 424–25.

"Health Report Interview with Professor Douglas Drossman: Irritable Bowel Syndrome." Radio National. www.abc.net.au. May 15, 2000.

"Irritable Bowel Syndrome." www.gihealth.com.

"Irritable Bowel Syndrome in Children." www.healing well.com.

"Irritable Bowel Syndrome: Treating the Mind to Treat the Body." *Tufts University Health and News Letter* 15 (September 1997): 4.

Kaye, Lisa, et al. "Irritable Bowel Syndrome: Which Definitions Are Consistent?" *Journal of the American Medical Association* 281 (February 17, 1999): 594.

"Lactose Intolerance FAQ." www.healingwell.com.

LaPook, Jonathan. "Irritable Bowel Syndrome (Colon Disorders)." In *Columbia University College of Physicians and Surgeons Complete Home Medical Guide,* 584. 3rd ed. New York: Columbia University, 1995.

Mann, Denise. "Yes, There Is a Cure for the Disease to Please." WebMD Medical News. www.onhealth. webmd.com. August 17, 2000.

Masand, Prakash S., Anthony J. Sousou, Sanjay Gupta, and David S. Kaplan. "Irritable Bowel Syndrome and Alcohol Abuse or Dependence." *American Journal of Drug and Alcohol Abuse* 24 (August 1998): 513.

Mathews, J. "In the Beast of the Belly: New Research Shows that Talk Therapy Helps Women with Irritable Bowel Syndrome." *Chatelaine* 72 (January 1999): 82.

McQuary, H. J., and R. A. Moore. "Antidepressants and Chronic Pain: Effective Analgesia in Neuropathic Pain and Other Syndromes." *British Medical Journal* 314 (March 15, 1997): 763.

McQuillan, Susan. "The 'Brain' Connection (Irritable Bowel Syndrome)." *American Health* 14 (September 1995): 64.

Medreview. "Irritable Bowel Syndrome FAQ." www.i-med review.com.

Missouri Arthritis Rehabilitation Research and Training Center. "Fibromyalgia FAQ." www.hsc.missouri.edu.

Mukherjee, M. "Disease to Please." www.emedlife.com. September 26, 2000.

Neal, K. R., J. Hebden, and R. Spiller. "Prevalence of Gastrointestinal Symptoms Six Months after Bacterial Gastroenteritis and Risk Factors for Development of Irritable Bowel Syndrome: Postal Survey in Patients." *British Medical Journal* 314 (March 15, 1997): 779.

Nicol, Rosemary. *Irritable Bowel Syndrome: A Natural Approach*. Berkeley, CA: Ulysses Press, 1999.

Pfasznik, Anne. "It's Not in Their Heads: IBS Sufferers Still Get Judged for Their Condition." *Journal of Addiction and Mental Health* May/June 2000, p. 1.

Pimental, M., M.D.; E. J. Chow, B.A.; and H. C. Lin, M.D. "Eradication of Small Intestinal Bacterial Overgrowth Reduces Symptoms of Irritable Bowel Syndrome." *American Journal of Gastroenterology* 95 (December 2000): 3503–06.

Reuters Health Information, London. "Novartis' Zelmac Shows Efficacy in Phase III Studies." http: www.gastro.org/reuters/2000/December/04/2000/28drgdoo3.html.

Rosenthal, M. Sara. *The Gastrointestinal Sourcebook*. Chicago: Contemporary Books/McGraw-Hill, 1997.

Salt, William B., M.D. *Irritable Bowel Syndrome and the Mind-Body-Brain-Gut Connection*. Columbus, Ohio: Parkview Publishing, 1997.

Selye, Hans. *The Stress of Life*. New York: McGraw-Hill, 1978.

Shimberg, Elaine F. *Relief from IBS*. New York: M. Evans & Co., 1988.

Sime, W. E. "Stress Management: A Review of Principles." www.unl.edu/stress/mgmt/.

"South American Tree Sap Is a Pain Killer, Anti-Inflammatory and Antibiotic." Natural Science Journal. http://www.natural science.com. May 15 2000.

Talley, Nichol J., M.D., Ph.D. "Treatment of Irritable Bowel Syndrome and Functional Constipation: New Insights." Report and transcripts of the Digestive Disease Week 2000 Seminar, Medscape.

Talley, N. J., S. E. Gabriel, and W. S. Harmsen. "Medical Costs in Community Subjects with Irritable Bowel Syndrome." *Gastroenterology* 109 (1995): 1736–41.

Taylor, Leslie. *Herbal Secrets of the Rainforest: The Healing Power of Over 50 Medicinal Plants You Should Know About.* Rocklin, Calif.: Prima Communications, 1998.

Taylor, M. L., D. R. Trotter, and M. E. Csuka. "The Prevalence of Sexual Abuse in Women with Fibromyalgia." *Arthritis and Rheumatism* 38 (1995): 229–34.

Toner, Brenda. "Irritable Bowel Syndrome Linked with Emotional Abuse." Center for the Advancement of Health. www.cfah.org.

Turnbull, G. K., M.D.; T. M. Vallis, Ph.D.; and D. Burstall, M.D. *IBS Relief: A Doctor, a Dietician and a Psychologist Provide a Team Approach to Managing Irritable Bowel Syndrome.* New York: John Wiley & Sons, 1998.

University of North Carolina. "Irritable Bowel Syndrome FAQ." www.med.unc.edu.

WebMD Medical News Staff. "FDA Warns Women with IBS about Drug's Severe Side Effects." http://my.web md.com. August 24, 2000.

"Women and Depression." www.psychologyinfo.com

"Women and Girls and Depression." www.wingsofmad ness.com

Yahoo!Health. "Depression FAQ." www.health.yahoo .com

Yahoo!Health. "Tai Chi FAQ." www.yahoo.com

"Yoga FAQ." www.yahoo.com

Index

acupuncture
  explained, 115
  finding reputable acupunc-
    turist, 115
acute and bacterial
  gastroenteritis
  and developing IBS, study,
    48–49
  explained, 48
Adams, Ansel, 102
alcohol abuse or dependence
  aperitif, 50
  depression as IBS trigger,
    50
  how it triggers IBS, 50–51
  and IBS, study, 50
  taking control, 51
Alcott, Louisa May, 107
alternative therapies
  acupuncture, 115
  biofeedback, 115–18
  Chinese herbal medicine
    (CHM), 111–14
  creative visualization,
    123–24
  hypnosis, 118–23
American Heritage
  Dictionary, 18

American Journal of Drug
  and Alcohol Abuse
  (August 1998), 49
American Journal of
  Gastroenterology
  (December 2000), 131
antibiotics
  bringing study to physi-
    cian's attention, 132
  and overabundant bacterial
    growth in IBS
    patients, study,
    131–32
antidepressants
  and IBS, how it works, 130
  as pain reliever, 130
  selective serotonin reuptake
    inhibitors (SSRIs),
    131
  tricyclic antidepressants
    (TCAs), 130–31
antidiarrheals, 133
antispasmodics
  (anticholinergic drugs)
  how often to use, 132
  for reducing painful
    colon spasms and
    cramping, 132

Barber Suggestibility Scale,
    The, 120–21
Beaumont, William
  about, 10–11
  (Experiments and Observa-
    tions on the Gastric
    Juice and the Physiol-
    ogy of Digestion), 11
  first to prove mind/gut
    connection, 11
biofeedback
  benefits to IBS sufferers,
    118
  explained, 116
  finding biofeedback
    practitioner, 118
  how it works, 117–18
  methods for monitoring
    different conditions,
    116–17
Blanchard, Edward, 28
body and mind connection
  depression, 24–30
  misinformed practitioners,
    17. *See also* doctors'
    attitudes
  stress, 17–24
British Medical Journal
    (March 15, 1997), 130

caffeine and IBS, 62–63
Chang, Lin, 33
Chatelaine (January 1999),
    95
chicken and other entrée take-
    out substitutions, 69

childhood, trying favorite
    activities from, 107–8
children with IBS, diet for
  older children, 74
  symptoms and treatment,
    73–74
Chinese food substitutions,
    69–70
Chinese herbal medicine
    (CHM)
  benefits for IBS sufferers,
    study, 112–14
  Bowel Symptom Scale, 113
  finding reputable herbalist,
    114
  origins, 111–12
  precautions, 114
chyme
  defined, 5
  in small intestine, 5–6
cognitive behavioral therapy
  catastrophizing, explained,
    29
  explained, 28–29
  significant reduction in
    IBS symptoms for
    patients undergoing,
    29
colectomy, 12
colon. *See* intestine, large
colon cancer
  annual physical, 13
  odds of developing, 12
  symptoms for seeking
    medical attention
    immediately, 13

constipation
  addressing discomfort
    of, 10
  defined, 9
  dietary patterns, lack of
    exercise, and not
    responding to urge, 9
  more serious causes of,
    9–10
conversion syndrome, 47
cramping and spasms,
  explained, 8
Creative Visualization
  (Gawain), 123
Crohn's disease
  explained, 12
  symptoms and
    treatment, 12
Croton lechleri, supplemental
    option
  Croton and pharmaceutical
    studies on, 128
  Croton vs. other antidiar-
    rheals, 128–29
  Provir (SP-303) trial
    studies for acute
    diarrhea, 128
  sangre de drago (blood of
    the dragon), uses, 127
  where to find, 129

dairy products triggering
  IBS, 61
delegating
  grocery shopping, ideas for,
    87–88

household chores, where to
    start, 87–88
  questions to ask
    yourself, 86
delicatessen substitutes
  breakfast, 67
  lunch, 68
depression
  as cause or effect of IBS,
    24–25
  distinguishing depression
    from other feelings,
    25–26
depression, therapy for
  brief psychodynamic
    therapy, 28
  catastrophizing, 29
  cognitive behavioral
    therapy, 29
  enteric nervous system, 30
  hypnosis, 29. *See also*
    hypnosis
  neurotransmitters, 30
  serotonin, 30
depression, types of
  dysthymia, 26–27
  major depression, 26
  manic-depressive illness, 27
  reactive depression, 27
diarrhea
  acute diarrhea, 8–9
  chronic conditions
    causing, 9
  chronic diarrhea, 9
  defined, 8
  nervous diarrhea, 9

diet diary, analyzing
  common trigger foods,
    60–63
  troublesome foods, pin-
    pointing, 63–64
diet strategies
  analyzing diet diary, 60–64
  diet for children with IBS,
    73–74
  fear of food, combating,
    75–76
  food allergies, 74–75
  food diary, keeping, 57–60
  making substitutions,
    65–72
  reintroducing foods into
    diet, 76–78
  right environment for
    eating, 72–73
digestive system (gastro-
    intestinal system), how
    it works
  large intestine, 6
  lumen and stomach, 5
  sensitivity to stress and
    strain, explained,
    19–20
  small intestine, 5–6
  upper GI tract and lower
    GI tract, 5
digestive system (gastro-
    intestinal system),
    problems with
  constipation, 9–10
  cramping and spasms, 8
  diarrhea, 8–9
  gas, 7–8

disease to please
  explained, 39
  how it affects IBS, 40
  learning to say no and
    managing, 40–41
  major factor contributing
    to, 39–40
  questions to ask yourself,
    41
  symptoms of, 39
  unhealthy relationships, 40
disorders linked with IBS
  functional disorders and
    IBS, 43–48
  physical disorders
    triggering IBS,
    48–54
diverticula, 13
diverticulitis, 13
diverticulum, 13
doctors' attitudes
  "IBS in American Women"
    (study), 33
  International Foundation
    for Functional
    Gastrointestinal
    Disorders, 33
  lack of understanding and
    effective treatment
    for, 32–33
  problem of uninformed
    doctors, 33
  taking control, 34
Drossman, Douglas, 23, 96
duodenum
  defined, 5–6
  how is works, 6

dyspepsia. *See* nonulcer
    dyspepsia
dysthymia, 26

eating, making mealtimes
    pleasant and positive,
    tips for, 72–73
emotional abuse and IBS
    self-blame, 36
    self-silencing, 36
environmental and job stress,
    20–21
exercise and stress
    exercise classes and
        workouts, 91
    explained, 88–89
    gardening, 91
    playing with children, 92
    tai chi chuan, 90–91
    walking, 92–95
    yoga, 89–90
Experiments and Observa-
    tions on the Gastric
    Juice and the Physiol-
    ogy of Digestion
    (Beaumont), 11

faith, finding help in
    house of worship, visiting,
        100–101
    talking with clergy, 100
fast-food substitutions
    breakfast, 65–66
    lunch and dinner, 66–67
fatigue and overwork
    as causes of stress, 21
    underlying factors, 21

fats triggering IBS, 60–61
fibromyalgia
    abnormality of deep sleep,
        44
    immune system changes, 45
    low levels of growth
        hormone, 44–45
    pain level of sufferers,
        43–44
    symptoms of, 43–44
    treatment for, 45
flatulence. *See* gas
food, combating fear of,
    75–76
    about, 75–76
    IBS triggers, 76
    when eating makes you
        sick, 76
food allergies
    determining, food reactions
        to consider, 52
    food extracts, 52
    reactions to, 51–52
    true allergy, explained, 51
food allergies, tests for
    determining
    determining food
        intolerance, 75
    radioallergosorbent test
        (RAST), 75
    scratch test, 74–75
food diary, keeping
    amount of liquid and foods
        involved, 59
    amounts eaten, 58–59
    behavior, don't alter during
        recording period, 58

circumstances for eating
    and drinking, 59
everything you eat and
    drink, 58
importance of, 57
keeping notebook, 60
logging notebook, 60
recording everything, 58
results of eating, 59–60
food intolerance, determining
    fructose, 53–54
    keeping food diary, 53
    lactose, 53
    sorbitol, 54
    wheat and wheat
        products, 53
foods, pinpointing
        troublesome eating
        habits, 64
    foods to eliminate, 63–64
    skipping meals altogether,
        64
foods, reintroducing in diet
    altering diet over period of
        time, 77
    BRAT diet for severe IBS,
        77
    expanding diet, 78
    food phobics, what to do,
        77
    foods comfortable to eat,
        noting, 78
    foods to begin with, 77–78
    reasons for eliminating
        trigger foods, 76–77
foods, triggering IBS
    caffeine, 62–63

dairy products, 61
fats, 60–61
high-fiber foods, 61–62
spices, 62
food substitutions
    chicken and other
        entrée takeout
        substitutions, 69
    Chinese food substitutions,
        69–70
    delicatessen substitutions,
        67–68
    fast-food substitutions,
        65–67
    home-cooked meal
        substitutions, 70–72
    Mexican food
        substitutions, 70
    pizza parlor substitutions,
        68
Frost, Robert, 102
fructose, 53–54

gardening for stress relief, 91
gas (flatulence)
    explained, 7
    foods high in undigestible
        carbohydrate, as
        cause of, 8
    how it occurs, 8
    swallowed air, as cause
        of, 7
    symptoms, 7
gastrointestinal system. *See*
    digestive system
Gawain, Shakti (*Creative
    Visualization*), 123

Gershon, Michael, 30
globus hystericus
  conversion syndrome,
    explained, 47
  explained, 47
  treatment, 47–48

*Harvard Group Scale of
  Hypnotic Susceptibility,
  The,* 121
Haye, Louise, 104
high-fiber foods triggering
  IBS, 61–62
home-cooked meal
  substitutions
  breakfast, 70–71
  dinner, 71–72
  lunch, 71
household chores, the disease
  to please, and stress
  delegating, 86–88
  explained, 85
humor for stress relief, 106
hypnosis
  explained, 119–20
  finding accredited
    professional, 122–23
  good candidates, tests for
    determining, 120–21
  hypnotic trance state, what
    to expect, 121–22
  potential for IBS relief, 122
  techniques for inducing, 121

IBS, diagnostic criteria for
  Manning criteria, 14

Rome criteria, 14–15
IBS and depression
  frustration and embarrass-
    ment, 24–25
  hopelessness, 24
  isolation, major factor in
    depression, 24
  other causes of depression,
    25
IBS and other stomach
    disorders
  colon cancer, 12–13
  diverticulitis, 13, 142
  inflammatory bowel disor-
    der (IBD), 12, 143
  understanding differences,
    11–12
IBS and sensitivity to stress
  excessive reaction of
    bowels of IBS
    sufferers, 23
  lower tolerance compared
    to general public, 23
IBS distress and mind/body
    connection
  Beaumont's observations
    on, 10–11
  importance of
    understanding, 11
  understanding IBS symp-
    toms as real physical
    reactions triggered
    by psychological
    factors, 11
ileum
  defined, 6
  function of, 6

inflammatory bowel disorder
  (IBD)
  Crohn's disease, 12
  IBD *vs.* IBS, 12
  ulcerative colitis, 12
internally generated stress, 20
intestine, large (colon)
  function of, 6
  motility, 6
  sections of, 6
intestine, small
  chyme. *See* chyme
  function of, 6
  ileocecal valve, 6
  sections of, 6
irritable bowel syndrome
  (IBS)
  defined, 4
  explained, 3
  factors triggering, 3–4
  functional disorder, 4
  symptoms, 3

jejunum
  defined, 5–6
  function of, 6
*Journal of Addiction and
  Mental Health*
  (May/June 2000),
  32, 33
*Journal of the American
  Medical Association*
  (JAMA), 112

lactose, 53
Lancet, The (January 20,
  1996), 48

Lao-tzu, 112
life's little irritants and stress,
  82–85
*Lion, the Witch, and the Ward-
  robe, The* (Lewis), 107
long-term stress
  physical symptoms of, 22
  psychological symptoms of,
    22
Los Angeles Time, 126
Lotronex fiasco
  approaching therapies
    cautiously, 127
  explained, 125–26
  medications and proactive
    behavior, 126–27

major depression, 26
manic-depressive illness
  defined, 26
  explained, 26–27
  symptoms of mania, 27
Manning criteria
  establishing IBS diagnosis,
    symptoms for, 14
  explained, 14
"Medical Costs in Commu-
    nity Subjects with
    Irritable Bowel
    Syndrome," 3
medications, over-the-counter
  Citrucel, Pepto Bismol, or
    Kaopectate for
    constipation, 133
  Pepcid and Beano for
    flatulence and
    cramping, 133

potential side effects
    exacerbating IBS,
    considering, 134
medication strategies
    antibiotics, 131–32
    antidepressants, 130–31
    antidiarrheals, 133
    antispasmodics, 132
    Croton lechleri, 127–29
    Lotronex fiasco, 125–27
    Zelmac and women with
        IBS, 129
menstrual cycle, effects of
    constipation and
        progesterone, 37–38
    increased bowel activity and
        prostaglandins, 38
    increased symptoms among
        IBS sufferers, 37
    recording symptoms, 37
    treatment for bowel
        disorders, 38, 39
Mesmer, Frank, 119
Mexican food
    substitutions, 70

nature, finding spiritual in
    other ways for enjoying
        nature, 102
    stress reduction
        opportunities, 101–2
    taking "nature break," 102
nonulcer dyspepsia
    drugs to avoid, 46
    dyspepsia, explained, 46
    IBS and dyspepsia, 47

nonulcer dyspepsia,
    explained, 46
    when to seek treatment, 46
Norton, Nancy, 33

Ornish, Dean, 89

physical disorders triggering
    IBS
    acute and bacterial gastro-
        enteritis, 48–49
    alcohol abuse or
        dependence, 49–51
    food allergies, 51–53
    food intolerance, 53–54
pizza parlor substitutions, 68
playing with children as stress
    reducer, 92
prayer and meditation,
    finding help through
    about, 103–4
    benefits of, 102–3
    sessions, scheduling, 105
    teaching yourself
        meditation, 104–5
psychodynamic therapy for
    depression
    explained, 28
    how it helps, 28
Psychosomatic Medicine
    (January/February
    2000), 36
psychotherapy and stress
    finding appropriate
        professional, 97–99
    gaining perspective with,
        95–96

improved self-worth, 96
practical therapy to look
    for, 99
questions for prospective
    therapist, 98–99
taking control over life and
    health, 96–97

reactive depression, 27
recommendations, goals for
    reading book
    important ideas, 2
    questions to ask yourself, 2
    what to look for while
        reading, 2
recommendations for apply-
    ing what you've learned
    addressing recurrence, 135
    benefits of improving life,
        135–36
    creating game plan, 133
    creating "time bank," 134
    don't get discouraged, 135
    including family and
        friends, 133–34
    loving food again, 134
    staying informed and trying
        something new,
        134–35
    tackling easiest recommen-
        dations first, 133
Reuters Health (November
    28, 2000), 127
Rome criteria
    establishing IBS diagnosis,
        factors for, 14–15
    explained, 14

self-blame, 36
self-silencing, 36
Selye, Hans
    coping with stress and
        well-being, 19
    developing first concept of
        stress, 18–19
    Stress of Life, 18
    subjectivity of stress, 79
sexual abuse in childhood and
    IBS
    cause-and-effect
        relationship
        between, 34
    emotional abuse and IBS.
        See emotional abuse
    fibromyalgia and chronic
        fatigue, 35–36
    other associations between,
        34–35
    and physical harm, 35–36
    reporting, stigma of, 34
short-term stress
    physical symptoms of, 21
    psychological symptoms
        of, 22
sorbitol, 54
spices and IBS, 62
spirituality and stress
    management
    faith, finding help in,
        100–101
    nature, finding spiritual in,
        101–2
    prayer and meditation,
        102–5
spiritual reminders, 108–10

St. Martin, Alexis
  about, 10
  subject of Beaumont's
      observations on
      stress and stomach
      problems, 10–11
Stanford Hypnotic
      Susceptibility Scales,
      The, 120
stomach
  chyme. *See* chyme
  defined, 5
  function of, 5
stress
  causes, 18
  defined, 18
  Hans Selye's concept of,
      18–19
  IBS and sensitivity to,
      22–23
  symptoms of, 18–19, 21–22
  types of, 19–21
stress, symptoms
  long-term stress, physical
      symptoms of, 22
  short- or long-term stress,
      psychological symp-
      toms of, 22
  short-term stress, physical
      symptoms of, 21
stress, types
  environmental and job
      stress, 20–21
  fatigue and overwork, 21
  gastrointestinal tract's
      sensitivity to stress,
      19

internally generated stress,
      20
  survival stress, 20
stress diary, keeping
  expectations of yourself,
      81
  how people affect you, 81
  what to track, 80–81
Stress of Life (Selye), 18
stressors, easily reduced
  household chores and
      disease to please, 85
  life's little irritants, 82–85
stressors, ranking and dealing
      with
  delegating, 86–88
  easily reduced, 82–85
stress-relievers, keeping close
  childhood activities,
      returning to favorite,
      107–8
  humor, 106
  spiritual reminders, 108–10
stress strategies
  benefits of journalizing,
      79–80
  keeping stress diary, 80–81
  psychotherapy and stress,
      95–99
  spirituality and stress
      management,
      99–105
  stress and exercise, 88–95
  stressors, ranking and
      dealing with, 82–88
  stress-relievers, keeping
      close by, 105–10

stress symptoms as cause of
stress
explained, 23
physical problems generat-
ing psychological
reactions, 23–24
survival stress, 20
Sweeting, Joseph, 24

tai chi chuan
benefits of, 90–91
classes, 91
Times, The, 126
Toner, Brenda, 32, 96
treatments and strategies for
managing IBS
affects of IBS, determining,
56
exhibiting symptoms established by Manning
or Rome criteria. *See*
Manning criteria and
Rome criteria
getting diagnosis, what to
expect, 55–56
keeping diet and stressors
diaries, 56
*Tufts University Health and
Nutrition Letter*
(September 1997),
27–28

ulcerative colitis
colectomy, 12
symptoms and treatment,
12

visualization, creative
affirmations, how they
help, 124
how it helps IBS sufferers,
123

walking
about, 92
calming benefits, how to
achieve, 93–95
wheat and wheat products,
53
Whitman, Walt, 102
women and IBS
disease to please, 39–42
doctors' attitudes, 32–34
IBS and childhood sexual
abuse, 34–37
"IBS in American
Women" (study),
31
menstrual cycle, effects of,
37–39
percentage affected by, 31

yoga
benefits of, 89
classes, what to expect,
89–90

Zelmac and women with IBS
for consitpation-
predominant
patients, 129
no benefits for men,
129